RESPITE CARE

Programs, Problems and Solutions

Edited by

Lynn M. Tepper, EdD
John A. Toner, EdD

The Charles Press, Publishers
Philadelphia

The Charles Press, Publishers
Post Office Box 15715
Philadelphia, PA 19103

Library of Congress Cataloging-in-Publication Data

Respite care: programs, problems and solutions / edited by Lynn M. Tepper
    and John A. Toner
        p. cm.
    Includes bibliographical references.
    ISBN 0-914783-67-X
    1. Respite care — United States. 2. Caregivers — United States.
I. Tepper, Lynn M.   II. Toner, John A.
    [DNLM: 1. Caregivers. 2. Respite Care.   WY 200 R4334 1993]
[HV1461.R474 1993]
362.1'0425 — dc20
DNLM/DLC
for Library of Congress   92-48396
                                                            CIP

Printed in the United States of America

ISBN 0-914783-67-X

The Charles Press acknowledges the American Institute of Life-Threatening Illness and Loss, a division of the Foundation of Thanatology.

Dedicated to my father, Jack Drukatz,
an impressive role model of successful
aging to all who know him.

L.M.T.

Dedicated to the memory of
Robert W. Toner, who taught his
children to love and be a respite to
one another, and to Brian, who has
learned the lesson well.

J.A.T.

Editors

Lynn M. Tepper, EdD
Director, Institute of Gerontology
Mercy College, Dobbs Ferry, New York
Associate Clinical Professor
Columbia University School of Public Health
New York, New York

John A. Toner, EdD
Assistant Professor of Clinical Public Health
Columbia University School of Public Health
Research Scientist, Department of Geriatrics
New York State Psychiatric Institute
New York, New York

Contributors

Virginia Barrett, DrPH
Research Scientist
Center for Geriatrics and Gerontology
Columbia University
The Hebrew Home for the Aged
New York, New York

Ronald S. Black, MD
Dementia Research Service
Burke Rehabilitation Institute
Cornell University Medical College
White Plains, New York

John Blass, MD
Dementia Research Service
Burke Rehabilitation Institute
Cornell University Medical College
White Plains, New York

JoAnn Canning, RN, CLU, ChFC
Senior Health Insurance Specialist
New York, New York

Carlo E. Grossi, MD
Director of Surgery
La Guardia Hospital
Forest Hills, New York

Carol Hegeman, MA
Director of Research
The Foundation for Long-Term Care
Albany, New York

Tamara Robin Jasper, MSW
Director, Herr Adult Day Center
Daughters of Israel Geriatric Center
West Orange, New Jersey

Terry Kinzel, MD, FACP
Clinical Professor of Medicine
Michigan State University
East Lansing, Michigan
Chief of Geriatrics and Gerontology
Veterans Affairs Medical Center
Iron Mountain, Michigan

Sandra Lewenson, EdD, RN
Assistant Professor of Nursing
State University of New York
Health Science Center at Brooklyn
Brooklyn, New York

Katherine Manning, BS, RN
Director, Northern Valley Adult Day Center
Community Centers for Mental Health, Inc.
Dumont, New Jersey

Theresa L. Martico-Greenfield, MPH
Assistant Director
The Jewish Home and Hospital for the Aged
New York, New York

Parathasarthy Narasinham, MD
La Guardia Hospital, H. I. P.
Forest Hills, New York

Karen Nolan, PhD
Dementia Research Service
Burke Rehabilitation Institute
Cornell University Medical College
White Plains, New York

Peter V. Rabins, MD
Associate Professor of Psychiatry
Johns Hopkins University School of Medicine
Baltimore, Maryland

Sally Robinson, DSW
Director, The Yonkers Office on Aging
Yonkers, New York

Gerald Rosner, CLU, ChFC
Insurance Specialist and Financial Planner
New York, New York

Elizabeth Ryan, RN
Dementia Research Service
Burke Rehabilitation Institute
Cornell University Medical College
White Plains, New York

Maura Ryan, PhD, RN, GNP
Director, Geriatric Nurse Practitioner Program
Hunter-Bellevue School of Nursing
New York, New York

Shura Saul, EdD, BCD, CSW
Educational Consultant
Kingsbridge Heights Health Care Facility
Bronx, New York
Adjunct Professor, School of Public Health
New York, New York

Sidney R. Saul, EdD, BCD, CSW
Psychotherapist
Goldensbridge, New York
Mental Health Consultant
Kingsbridge Heights Health Care Facility
Bronx, New York

Pamela Schneider, MSW, CSW
Associate Executive Director for Programs,
VISIONS Services for the Blind
and Visually Impaired
New York, New York

Joyce Storey, BSN, MSEd, RN
Administrative Nursing Supervisor
Operating Room Consultant
Montefiore Medical Center
New York, New York

Mayra Suero-Wade, DDS, MPH
President, Dentistry in Motion
Dumont, New Jersey
Dentist in private practice
New York, New York

Lynn M. Tepper, EdD
Director, Institute of Gerontology
Mercy College, Dobbs Ferry, New York
Associate Clinical Professor
Columbia University School of Public Health
New York, New York

Jeanne A. Teresi, PhD
Research Associate
The Hebrew Home for the Aged
Research Scientist
Center for Geriatrics and Gerontology
Columbia University
New York, New York

John A. Toner, EdD
Assistant Professor of Clinical Public Health
Columbia University School of Public Health
Research Scientist, Department of Geriatrics
New York State Psychiatric Institute
New York New York

Margaret Traher, MS, RN
Dementia Research Service
Burke Rehabilitation Institute
Cornell University Medical College
White Plains, New York

Nancy D. Weber, MSSW, ACSW
Executive Director
VISIONS Services for the Blind
and Visually Impaired

Audrey S. Weiner, MPH
Director, Mental Health
The Jewish Board of Family and
Children's Services
New York, New York

Contents

Caregiver Concerns

Respite Care Research

Preface

Anyone who assumes the duties and primary responsibilities of caregiver for an elderly relative or other chronically disabled family member soon learns that the caregiver's role is often overwhelming, adversely affecting even the most compassionate samaritan. In most family situations the caregiver must be in attendance almost constantly, ready to respond to the unrelenting needs of parents, spouses, children or other relatives who are unable to care for themselves. The job is essentially constant, never-ending, tragic to experience and, not infrequently, a thankless effort. Consider the physical stress the family caregiver faces each and every day while caring, for example, for an elderly parent with Alzheimer's disease, a husband totally unable to care for himself because of the complete disability caused by amyotrophic lateral sclerosis, or a 14-year-old son with muscular dystrophy, kept alive solely with a respirator.

How common are these problems and how often is respite care needed? It is estimated that 15 percent of persons over the age of 60 require some form of long-term care. To this huge number must be added children and young adults with severely disabling conditions who must be cared for at home for prolonged periods.

It is hardly surprising that caregivers develop burnout along with physical and psychological problems so that they themselves ultimately require help. This help may be in the form of respite care, in other words, *care for the caregiver*.

Within the past few years the concept of respite care has assumed an important role in the continuum of long-term care and is now recognized as a key component of caregiving programs for the elderly and disabled. Simply stated, unless the caregiver is functioning effectively, the other elements of care suffer greatly and may in turn have reduced value.

Although there are several different approaches to respite care, all have the same basic objective: to provide caregivers with temporary, intermittent, substitute care, allowing for relief from the daily responsibilities of caring for the elderly or disabled. Respite care is essential for all caregivers, whether they are formal providers (who work for an institution) or informal providers (family members or close friends).

This book describes respite care in detail: what it is; how it functions; practicalities of implementation; and problems involved in its solution. Models of institutional and community-based respite care are presented to familiarize the reader with a typology of respite care, as well as benefits, drawbacks and cost to the consumer. As crucial elements in the quality of respite services, operational viability, considerations related to marketing, recruitment, training and case management are discussed. Also included are separate chapters devoted to recently developed models of adult day care, hospice care, in-home care and specific programs for in-home dental care, dementia patients and the visually impaired. As with any new and evolving movement, many different issues must be addressed. *Respite Care: Programs, Problems and Solutions* identifies both the programmatic and caregiver barriers to respite care — financial, medical, personal and social.

In this book a case study approach has been used to illustrate the more typical conditions and situations surrounding caregiving. This gives the contributing authors the opportunity to describe the actual concerns of families and the people they care for, as well as the ability to describe innovative approaches to caregiving. Caregiver concerns are also emphasized throughout the book. A historical look at caregiving will help readers to understand the evolution of respite care. Caregiving to individuals with cancer is discussed from a multidisciplinary perspective because the needs for respite care are similar yet different from caregiving to those with other chronic conditions.

No approach to the subject of respite care is complete without examples of recent research initiatives, so critical to the development, implementation and evaluation of this type of care. We cannot determine that respite services have met their stated goals of improving caregiver well-being, reducing institutionalization and reducing the cost of care without measuring the effectiveness of programs to achieve these and other goals.

To be successful, respite care must include representatives of many disciplines such as nursing, medicine, social work, psychiatry, psychology, dentistry and administration, among others. These respective contributions to respite care are described throughout the book.

This book represents the first time in a single volume that respite care has been examined in full detail. It is likely that much more will be forthcoming about this most important form of long-term care.

Models of Respite Care

1

Models of Institutional and Community-Based Respite Care

Carol Hegeman, MA

There are many types of geriatric respite programs and sponsors. Geriatric respite is provided by groups, agencies and various different types of institutions. Locations of service are equally varied—from within elders' homes, to community settings, to many kinds of elder care institutions and hospitals.

In a national study done by the Foundation for Long-Term Care (FLTC) in 1987,* five major types of geriatric respite care delivery were found. In this chapter these different types and some of their possible variants are described. After a brief typology of programs, there is a case study of a program typifying each mode, followed by a discussion of the benefits and drawbacks of each model in terms of caregiver/elder benefits, cost and operational viability. Following the discussion of each model, current (1993) costs are presented.

A TYPOLOGY OF RESPITE MODELS

The major types of geriatric respite in 1987 were:

1. In-home respite (provided by special respite agencies, home care agencies, and by general community agencies)

---

* There have not been any more recent studies of this magnitude. The results, where possible, have been updated to reflect current costs.

2. Respite provided in community settings (adult day care providers, freestanding respite facilities and respite care cooperatives)
3. Institutions caring for the elderly (senior housing, continuing care retirement communities, adult homes and nursing homes)
4. Hospitals (VA and community)
5. Combination groups comprised of two or more of the above

None of these types is monolithic. There are differences in fees and financing, use of staff and volunteers, and even in mission and definition within each group. Some operate under state demonstration programs, others seemed to bloom where they were serendipitously seeded. Some successful models seem to share little in common with others except a fierce determination by program managers to serve caregivers and elders successfully. Other programs group together to form coherent patterns.

IN-HOME RESPITE

In the study conducted by the Foundation for Long-Term Care, 15 percent of respondents offered in-home respite exclusively and another 6 percent offered in-home respite in conjunction with one or more respite models, most typically a nursing home/in-home combination.

Benefits and Drawbacks to Consumers

In-home respite is inherently appealing when care outside the home would be physically or emotionally difficult for the elder, for example, when the caregiver negatively perceives out-of-home care. Disruption of the day-to-day routine is minimized when the respite worker literally replaces the caregiver in her own home. A diligent respite agency representative can advise how to make the home situation more suited to long-term care and during a medical assessment, can possibly identify untreated problems.

For caregivers leaving for an extended period of time, however, the one-to-one replacement model may seem frightening. They may be afraid that the respite worker will not show up or do the job correctly and diligently. While all competent home care and respite programs do indeed provide promised coverage, caregiver anxiety may remain. In-home respite also puts a tremendous burden on the respite worker to provide sustained substitute care. When the worker and elder are compatible, in-home respite can be an enriching experience for both. If they are not, the quality of care may suffer. The variety of caregivers that are in other kinds of settings may be a form of protection from a caregiver who does not mesh well with the person they are caring for.

Costs

In 1987, the cost of in-home respite varied from $2.35 an hour to $7 an hour with a mean cost of $4.26. In 1993, this service costs $5.03 to $12.40 per hour. Per diem costs in 1987 ranged from $15 to $70 with a mean cost of $42. These costs were lower than skilled nursing facility (SNF) and hospital costs, at a mean of $76 and $66, respectively, but also may well reflect a lower level of care.

Eighty-one percent of in-home programs accepted no Medicaid at all. For all survey respondents, 57 percent accepted no Medicaid-eligible respite clients. If a patient is Medicaid-eligible, institutional care may be less expensive.

Operational Viability

Nineteen percent of all in-home respite programs reported showing a profit. This percentage is slightly higher than the 13 percent of the other survey respondents who reported showing a profit. Another 31 percent of in-home programs reported breaking even financially. This percentage, too, is slightly higher than the 24 percent of all other survey respondents who reported breaking even.

A major problem facing home care is the unavailability of personnel. Although the shortage of staff affects all long-term care, finding in-home respite workers can be especially difficult, but exactly how difficult seemed to vary among programs. The case study of INTERAC shows possible strategies for staff recruitment.

One model of in-home respite providing an innovative source of workers for in-home respite is Project Time-Out, developed by the Center for Intergenerational Learning, Institute of Aging, at Temple University. This model program trains college students as temporary in-home respite workers for impaired elders. Students are matched, trained and supervised by staff of the Center for Intergenerational Learning and paid directly by the families that used their services.

Another problem for home care in general and for in-home respite in particular is quality assurance when there is no on-site supervisor present.

Case Study A: An In-Home Respite Model

INTERAC, a nonprofit, community-based human services agency serving a cohesive working-class community in Philadelphia, offers geriatric respite care in elders' own homes for a few hours or a few days. Like many home-based programs, its "respite" component is similar to its regular services. Its program, in its fourth year of operation in 1987, had a yearly budget of $102,000 and a typical daily caseload of 25 clients. Six years later, in 1993, the yearly budget has more than doubled to $215,000 and the daily typical caseload has risen to 40 clients daily. It was chosen as a case study because it operates at a modest profit (only 19 percent of similar programs show a profit) and it showed unusual creativity in developing clients, workers and financial support.

Recruitment and Admission

Aggressive marketing proved effective after a slow first year. Most successful were the newspaper features and articles, although traditional outreach activities of brochures and speaking engagements also were important. As of this writing, demand for the service matches the supply of workers.

As with many other home-based agencies, however, recruiting and retaining workers proves more difficult than recruiting clients. The problem of recruitment at INTERAC is how to attract and retain respite workers on a pay scale varying in 1987 from $3.88 per hour for homemaker services to $4.69 per hour for home health aides. The pay scale in 1993 varies from $5.03 per hour for homemaker services to $7.57 for home health aides. No benefits are provided.

In the program's early years, a part-time respite management team consisting of a public health nurse and a marketing/business manager developed a series of labor retention strategies that capitalized on the workers' desire for local, gratifying work. Free Red Cross training on geriatric care was provided. Dress codes underscored the professionalism this training provided. Weekly meetings with supervisors developed collegial skills and a sense of belonging to the organization that is traditionally a missing element in part-time aide work. Workers could choose the number of hours they worked, as well as the families they worked with; the opportunity to work with clients on a continuing basis was offered whenever possible.

Workers came to the INTERAC offices weekly to pick up their paychecks and the respite management team used this time for individual supportive sessions in which respite workers' concerns could be addressed. This again underscored the agency's strong effort to create a sense of belonging.

While admission is open to all elders at INTERAC, they often are screened by INTERAC's service management system, particularly when multiple problems are evident. This type of case management appears to be a crucial element in the quality of respite services: it allows respite to be used appropriately; it allows for the provision of other needed services; and it avoids overuse or misuse of services. The nurse coordinator matches elders to clients, reviews the care plan and follows workers reports on their clients. The patients that are eligible for this service must be medically stable however, confused and/or incontinent patients are handled routinely. A signed contract is required, specifying the length of the respite stay, the level of care that will be given, the charge for the service and who will pay.

Respite Operations

The most striking feature of this particular respite service is the close involvement and concern of the supervisory staff for the program. Like many successful social service programs, sound and creative management combine with an unusually deep staff commitment to the project. An attempt to match workers' personalities and skills with an appropriate respite client adds a "homey" quality to this respite service that simply would not be possible in a larger, more impersonal agency.

The program has undergone many changes since inception: staff turnover at the management level; dropping the idea of a volunteer cadre of workers (it proved infeasible); and adding a sliding payment scale with a reduced fee for eligible clients.

Scheduling visits with appropriate workers is handled by a respite care coordinator in conjunction with the case management service also managed by INTERAC when deemed necessary. The use of this existing case management mechanism ensures that respite can become part of a long-term care system instead of an isolated "bandaid" approach to a complex problem. The case management approach keeps utilization appropriate as well. Clients who have needs other than respite can be referred to other services such as INTERAC's adult day care program.

Training for staff that was once conducted by the Red Cross is now done by alternative methods. Private instructors proved very expensive. Existing hospital training programs to which workers were sent proved cheaper and quite satisfactory.

Quality assurance is always a problem in a home-care delivery system, where actual day-to-day observation is impossible. Share-the-Care relies on training, weekly meetings with staff and on-site visits by the respite nurse to assure that quality care is delivered. Other quality assurance mechanisms include scheduled discussion time with aides, random telephone checks to elders and caregivers, home visits by supervisory staff and regular staff evaluation.

Perhaps the most interesting aspect of this respite service has been the mix of revenues it relies on to bring it to financial stability. The program was started by grants of $75,000 for operations and $15,000 for developing a marketing and business plan. In 1987, revenues from service yielded about $1.30 an hour more than actual cost of the service. In 1993, the profit yielded by this organization is about $1.43 an hour. The 1993 average national figures for in-home care are: $8 an hour for homemaker services; $10 an hour for a 2-hour visit and $9 per hour for the cost of 3 or 4 hours of a home health aide; $90 per day on weekends and $100 per day on weekends for live-in home health aides. An expansion into providing contractual home care services for an area hospital generates additional income to sustain the respite project. Attempts at lowering costs through a volunteer program, however, were not successful.

COMMUNITY-BASED RESPITE: ADULT DAY CARE AND FREESTANDING PROGRAMS

Community-based respite programs represented 41 percent of all survey respondents. These include adult day care programs and freestanding respite facilities. Adult day care services were frequently offered by an institutional site or as part of a spectrum of respite services. Adult day care respite will be discussed first, followed by a brief discussion of freestanding respite facilities. Another model that belongs in this category is the respite co-op, the case study used for this model.

Benefits and Drawbacks to Consumers

Adult day care respite programs are usually regular adult day care programs that keep several slots open to allow an unscheduled "drop in" service for elders when their caregivers need a break. Some adult day care programs consider their entire operation as "ongoing respite," but this definition diminishes the uniqueness of the respite concept. Such a routine service seems to be part of a formal array of elder care services and avoids the challenge of the truly excellent respite program: caring simultaneously for the elder, the caregiver and the caregiver-elder unit.

Adult day care-based respite offers an excellent option for caregivers who need respite for less than 8 hours. Most out-of-home services are often available only for days at a time. The day care concept is an excellent option for elders who would enjoy the stimulation of group activities and the chance for conversation with peers. If the elder has been understimulated at home, the adult day care center may be far more satisfying than when an aide comes to the home. A typical problem with adult day care is transportation. The elder must be transportable by car, or the adult day care center must provide a van able to accommodate nonambulatory patients.

Like most good respite programs, adult day programs should, through an initial assessment, provide a professional overview of the client and suggest adjustments to the day-to-day routine at home that may improve care.

The survey yielded three freestanding respite services: one that operates a separate barrier-free apartment set up on the grounds of a hospital/nursing home; a respite service run for both the elderly living with family and the elders in need of emergency housing; and one in a hospital-based hospice. The advantage common to all programs is that they offer a secure, well-supervised, out-of-home program where the caregiver's or the elder's do not perceive the stay as an institutionalization.

Costs

In 1987, adult day care costs averaged $3.75 per hour and $43.63 per diem. According to the National Council on Aging's 1989 census, these rates ranged from $3 to $150 per day, with an average rate of $34 per diem. The freestanding program, combined respite and emergency housing, costs $32 per diem. The two other freestanding programs charge no fees.

Operational Viability

One freestanding program found in the FLTC survey—the no-charge, barrier-free apartment—was operating at 100 percent occupancy after only 6 months: 33 percent of funding was from a grant; the other 66 percent came from the hospital/nursing home sponsor. The second ran at about 75 percent occupancy and was not self-sufficient. The hospice program also ran at a loss and was subsidized by the sponsoring hospital.

It certainly seems that freestanding programs appeal to outside sponsors. Adult day programs offer respite in conjunction with other regular services, so there are few separate operational issues inherent in the respite component itself.

Case Study B: A Family Respite Co-op Model

In the family respite co-op model, an existing adult day health care program operates a weekend respite program using paid staff augmented by unpaid workers who are caregivers of participating elders. These caregivers trade a unit of work at the co-op for four units of free weekend respite. The Family Respite Co-op of Sacramento was chosen for a case study because it is unique in its concept, its hours of operation and its adjunct services. This case study, unlike all the others, was conducted by telephone and not in person.

Program Description

The Family Respite Co-op is open from 9 a.m. to 9 p.m. on Saturdays and from 9 a.m. to 5 p.m. on Sundays. It operates from the Rosenwald C. Robertson Adult Day Health Care Center, which is only open weekdays. Twenty-seven elders are enrolled in the co-op, but the average daily attendance is eight. The program maintains a ratio of one caregiver to four clients. Two paid staff, a half-time respite coordinator and a full-time LVN (licensed vocational nurse) are on duty at all times. Family caregivers augment these professionals. Daily activities are similar to many social day care programs. Meals are simple brown-bag affairs that are brought by the family but eaten together family style. Nonmembers of the co-op (those caregivers who choose not to trade time for respite) may also use the respite service on a fee-for-service basis. They pay $25 a day or $5 an hour for weekend respite.

The Respite Co-op is unusual in several ways. First, through an as-yet-untested arrangement with neighboring Hillhaven Nursing Home, it will provide a weekend "bed and breakfast" respite. In this option, a family will arrange for a full weekend of respite. The elder will be brought to the co-op on Saturday morning. On Saturday evening, a respite staff member will escort the elder to Hillhaven where a special respite bed is waiting. After breakfast at Hillhaven, the elder will be returned to spend Sunday at the Respite Co-op. Whether such multiple movement back and forth will be too disorienting for elders is a valid question that will simply have to be tested by time.

Second, the co-op maintains a registry of in-home caregivers who have been screened by the co-op (but neither bonded nor employed by them) in conjunction with a local geriatric nurse. This registry is provided as a service to home caregivers who wish to use a home-based service as well as to people merely calling for information on existing services.

Finally, participation in the Respite Co-op for families who can neither donate time to work nor pay for services is made possible by a linkage with a local college fraternity. Fraternity members provide a minimum of 3 hours a week of caregiving service.

Recruitment and Admission

When this program began in February 1987, the co-op sponsor, Rosen-wald C. Robertson Adult Day Health Care Center, undertook a classic marketing campaign. News releases and brochures were developed and disseminated; a speakers' bureau targeted senior citizens' groups, churches, women's clubs, community services, social service agencies and business and civic groups. Paid advertising was used in small community newspapers. In retrospect, the respite coordinator feels that the market-ing effort was hampered by trying to introduce two relatively new con-cepts—respite and cooperatives—simultaneously. Each concept needed introduction and explanation. Were she to begin her marketing anew, the concept of weekend respite care would have been marketed first. Once the respite concept was more familiar, the optional co-op method of participation would be introduced. Current marketing takes this tack. The current co-op membership of 27 caregiver/elder units is too small for the co-op to be self-sufficient. A second marketing campaign to increase membership and encourage fee-for-service use is planned.

Admission requirements are loose. Participants are rejected only if they are bedridden, in the later stages of Alzheimer's disease, or if their attendance compromises the safety or welfare of other participants. Almost all clients suffer from some sort of dementia. Doors are chimed to ring when opened, so wanderers are protected, especially since the enrollment and caregiver/elder ratio remains low.

A "free care" day for potential participants allows potential client behavior to be reviewed. It also provides a no-risk overview of the program for caregivers. The admission process begins when the caregivers of a prospective client return a completed application form. Emergency plans, medical status, and behavioral characteristics are all reviewed prior to the "free care" day. If the data on the application form and the respite client's behavior during the free care day meet program requirements, the client is accepted. There is no home visit.

Management Strategies

The activities at the Respite Co-op are kept simple. No professional physical therapist or activities director is on duty during the weekend period. Gardening, bingo, movies and general conversation are main activities. Most clients tend to stay for one 3-hour unit, encompassing one meal, free socialization and an activity.

A major challenge for the respite coordinator is managing the respite co-op caregiver-volunteer. Each volunteer must take a 3-hour class

on physical care techniques. Once trained, the volunteer must be scheduled into one of twenty-eight 3-hour slots each 4-week period. Volunteers
usually choose to work at the beginning or the end of the care period for
their elder. This strategy avoids a double trip to the center.

Of the 27 participants enrolled at the center, only four are enrolled
on a fee-for-service basis. Increasing the number of clients who pay for
services presents a "Catch-22" type of challenge to the respite co-op
concept. On one hand, it expands the revenue base. On the other, it
erodes the co-op concept itself. Presently, the county welfare department
is exploring a contract for Saturday respite that might produce the
revenue needed to keep the co-op financially stable.

Management issues for the "bed and breakfast" option are worked
out on paper, but are as yet untested in practice. Arrangements will need
to be made the week before the weekend admission. Admission to the
nursing home will depend upon room availability, ability to pay the
regular skilled nursing facility rate privately and the respite client's status.
The client will need to be continent and be able to ambulate independently.

The registry service of home respite workers is managed informally,
in sharp contrast to the formal aide services of INTERAC and the
Metropolitan Commission on Aging (case studies A and E). It is a simple
referral service with no formal endorsement or management of home
workers when hired. Aides choosing to register are often former Respite
Co-op members whose elders are now either deceased or institutionalized. The Respite Co-op manager notes that geriatric care is often the one
marketable skill some former caregivers possess and that the professionalism of a previously unpaid occupation can provide a new sense of
empowerment, often leading to further education and a new "career."

Whether this novel concept will eventually be self-supporting is an
important issue that will only be answered with time. With its creative use
of caregivers and unused space, it offers new areas for development and
innovation in respite care.

RESPITE IN INSTITUTIONS: CARING FOR THE ELDERLY

Geriatric respite care is being provided, in decreasing order of frequency
according to the 1987 survey, by skilled nursing facilities (40 percent),
intermediate care facilities (31 percent), adult homes (17 percent) and
senior housing (4 percent).

Benefits and Drawbacks to Consumers

Despite major differences in the functional levels of respite clients they can serve, skilled nursing facilities (SNFs), intermediate care facilities (ICFs) and adult homes share certain benefits for caregivers and elders seeking respite.

First, continual care is assured. Oversight of the elder does not rest, as it does in home care, on one aide who must wait until the replacement aide arrives before leaving. This element of certainty is ideal for a caregiver who is without nearby relatives and who wishes to take a vacation away from home. Peace of mind may be enhanced further by the medical staffing of the nursing home models. Other families who are uneasy with the thought that strangers are in their home may prefer to move their elderly relative to an institution.

Second, the move may be perceived as advantageous for elders as well. For mentally intact elders, a respite stay in an exemplary institution may prove to be a needed vacation from home. All nursing homes and adult homes in the survey provide recreational, social and ancillary services (such as hairdressing and religious services) that are not easily available to a house-bound elder. Some providers report that some respite patients, in fact, catalyze permanent residents to participate in activities, saying, in essence, that all these opportunities are not to be taken for granted. Some respite programs capitalize on this benefit and market themselves as "vacation days."

Third, in some cases the medical work-up that is part of a nursing home stay may result in a change in a drug regimen or diet that can have positive health benefits. This improvement most often occurs when a patient is not receiving any formal services at home. This lack of services was reported for 29 percent of respite clients.

The downside of this equation is that some elders and caregivers will regard institutional placement as unacceptable. An elder may simply refuse to leave the home. A caregiver may feel the move will be too upsetting for the elder and the caregiver therefore feels too guilt-ridden. If these feelings cannot be modified, the institutional option, no matter how objectively appealing to an outside case manager or friend, may be inappropriate.

As discussed earlier, there have been studies of the effects of institutional respite on the frail elderly. Prior to these studies, a common assumption was that the phenomenon of "transfer trauma" might cause permanent mental and physical deterioration or even death. An earlier study by the FLTC analyzed the health status of 137 frail elders one month after an institutional respite stay. Of these elders, 51 percent were reported to be unchanged by the visit; 21 percent were reported worse; and a surprising 26 percent were reported improved (Perdue 1984). Another study indicated that the majority of respite recipients either displayed no change in function or that there had been positive changes (Scharlach and Frenzel 1986).

One benefit of institutional respite commonly reported by providers is that while respite is intended to delay institutionalization as long as possible, it greatly softens the blow of permanent institutionalization when it does occur. Respite visits engender a positive relationship between elder, caregiver, and facility staff, leading to a smoother transition and less feelings of guilt for the family.

A caveat seems in order here: a smooth transition to placement is certainly not the purpose of a respite stay and any attempt to encourage permanent placement when home care is still a viable option seems to subvert the entire respite concept. Yet the frailty of the population served in respite does mean that eventual institutionalization may be inevitable. When that occurs, reduced stress can only be seen as a positive component of the service.

Costs

Institutional respite care costs varied from an average, in 1987, of $44.11 per diem in adult homes, $66.99 per diem in ICFs and $76.39 per diem in SNFs. Six years later in 1993, daily rates have increased by 67% to $197 per day. Medicaid was accepted by 39 percent of SNFs, 26 percent of ICFs and 23 percent of adult homes.

Operational Viability

The case study of St. John's Nursing Home Visiting Resident Days provides operational detail. Several factors, while not universally true for all models of this type, are common and significant enough to note here. Four common factors are: limited bed availability; the need to avoid caregiver attempts to use respite to subvert the regular admission process; minimum length-of-stay requirements; and difficulty in providing respite on an emergency basis.

About 36 percent of elder care institutional programs in our survey offer respite on a "bed-available" basis; that is, if a bed on a regular unit is empty at the time of the respite query, the respite placement is possible. If a call is received when no bed is available or an attempt is made to reserve a bed for respite in advance, that request simply cannot be honored. If respite is to be an integral part of a long-term care delivery system, this "maybe" system of bed availability will not work.

The reasons that facilities are unwilling to set aside a bed are primarily financial. Because of huge waiting lists in many states for nursing home placement, it is easy to match a long-term care bed with a permanent resident and have the income for that bed be assured. Nationally, SNF beds set aside for respite had an occupancy rate of only 52 percent. At an average SNF rate of about $76 per diem, one set-aside bed at the national occupancy rate can cost a facility $13,315 in foregone revenue per year. Strategies are discussed in later chapters for increasing the overall SNF occupancy rate. However, facilities that would like to offer respite but cannot afford the probable loss of revenue need to take their dilemma to policymakers.

ICFs and adult homes tend to have a higher percentage of unused beds and thus would be ideal locations for respite beds. Ironically, however, respite is needed most at the SNF level. Usage at the ICF and adult program level is extremely low. Adult homes report only a 33 percent usage rate for their respite beds, ICFs only 49 percent occupancy.

In a study done by Home Aides of Central New York, out of 338 institutional respite referrals made over 5 years, 229 referrals were to the SNF level, 16 to the ICF level and 23 to the adult home level. In the FLTC's own respite programs operating in New York State's Capital District, a similar skewing of respite placement toward skilled nursing facility level was noted. Such low usage makes ICF and adult home respite viable only if the programs are a part of a multifaceted respite program.

Another factor that affects the operation of an institutionally based respite program is the need to assure that respite beds are indeed used for respite and not as a short cut to a permanent long-term care bed. Management strategies to avoid such misuse are described in detail in the St. John's case study. Because the possibility for misuse is always present, institutional respite may not be appropriate for families who have decided to permanently place their elder and are waiting for an available bed. This kind of respite user seems more likely to misuse respite than does a family committed to home care and seeking a break. Accordingly, some institutional providers have established a policy to steer families seeking permanent nursing home placement away from respite and toward home care support.

Still another operational roadblock is put up by paperwork and medical screening needed at admission. Because paperwork requirements often equal permanent admission, few nursing homes take respite recipients for less than two weeks. This requirement leaves a gap in respite provision. Home-based respite and community-based respite are focused on short caregiver absences; institutional and hospital-based respite are geared toward long caregiver absences. People seeking respite for 2 to 12 days may not be able to find it easily.

A significant operational characteristic that distinguishes institutional respite from other models is that it cannot usually handle respite requests quickly. A typical admission is scheduled in advance, as the bed often needs to be reserved. Critical elements, such as a home visit, a physical examination, and a means test for Medicaid, must be completed prior to admission. Although these requirements are necessary to assure high-quality care, they act to keep emergency respite placements out of institutions.

Case Study C: A Home Visiting Resident Program

St. John's Home, a multilevel, multiservice nursing home in Rochester, New York, has offered an institutional respite care program at the skilled nursing facility (SNF) level for 5 years. These years of experience have combined with strong community linkages to enable the facility to develop respite management strategies that both optimize benefits to clients and maximize operational efficiency. Although no one element of the respite program may be unique to St. John's Home, the impressive combination of exemplary respite provision and well-thought-out management strategies make this program an ideal model for new or developing institutional respite programs.

Program Description

St. John's Home offers two private SNF rooms for respite stays for 1 to 6 weeks. In 1987, the daily fee was $119. Thirty-six percent of payments are private pay; the balance, 64 percent, is billed to Medicaid. The beds are set aside exclusively for respite usage. St. John's Home had a 1987 occupancy rate of 98.8 percent, an impressively high percentage when compared to an average rate of 53 percent in the FLTC's national respite study. Staff is specifically assigned to respite cases, although no one works exclusively with respite. Sixty-five percent of respite clients at St. John's are repeat clients.

Recruitment and Admission

Although respite is marketed in all publicity efforts, staff reports that "word of mouth" is the primary source of referral. Initially, television and newspapers proved to be the most effective marketing media. The availability in Rochester of integrated case management for all Medicaid patients (ACCESS) that routinely refers clients to the St. John's respite program is undoubtedly a positive contributor to this high occupancy rate. Referrals through this system become ongoing and easier.

The admissions process usually requires lead time of two to three months. One admissions representative is responsible for helping clients fulfill admission requirements. A home visit, a firm discharge plan, a detailed social and medical report, and a plan for financial arrangements are all required prior to admission. Medicaid patients need approval by the appropriate agency; private-pay patients must pay before admission. The admissions representative also maintains a "back-up" reservation list of people who can use respite on short notice if there is a cancellation.

The home visit is a crucial component of the admission process. The goals of the visit are to determine the medical and social needs of the proposed respite client, as well as to determine the motivation for the stay by the caregiver. Clients who do not meet the criteria for a respite stay are referred elsewhere.

One type of client is always inappropriate for a respite stay: When the usual caregiver is looking not for temporary relief from care, but rather for a way—consciously or unconsciously—to get the elder admitted to the nursing home by attempting to use respite to circumvent the extensive waiting list for permanent admission, the respite coordinator should take notice. The home visit, therefore, is used for more than the usual patient assessment to determine level of care and treatment plans. It becomes a way for the respite care staff to determine the caregiver's motivation for the stay and to make referrals to appropriate services for clients who are really seeking or who need permanent long-term care placement.

The home-visit team at St. John's consists of a social worker and registered nurse who closely observe not only the potential respite recipient but also the respite unit—caregiver and care recipient. Certain behavior and attitudes should trigger probing questions: lack of communication between caregiver and elder, lack of honesty about the visit, "house-for-sale" signs that indicate a possible permanent move, or indefinite vacation plans. No respite client is ever admitted if the social worker and RN are not confident that the respite recipient will be able to return home. When the caregiver appears uncertain about discharge plans, the team refers the clients to other community services.

The home visit also provides important preliminary data for a care plan and assures that the expectations of both caregiver and elder are appropriate. Appropriate client wishes for the care plan are carefully followed. Some caregivers want a respite stay that primarily ensures safety. Others want to replicate as closely as possible the conditions at home. Still others envision the stay as a "vacation," providing an enriching, invigorating experience for an elder who lacks stimulation at home. Since both caregivers and care recipients are the clients served by respite, a care plan must be designed to meet reasonable expectations, to benefit the elder, and to make the return home as smooth as possible.

To illustrate why the respite team is so careful about designing a care plan with both clients in mind, the St. John's staff cites an example in which an aggressive care plan designed to rehabilitate the respite recipient could work against the combined well-being of the unit. It involves a respite stay for a wheelchair-bound elder who could be ambulated successfully with physical therapy and the assistance of nursing aides. Once this client returned home, however, continued ambulation was impossible, because his only caretaker, his wife, was herself too frail to assist him. Unless the wife would allow the hiring of an aide to assist her husband in walking, the stress engendered by the change in the demands of care at home could be destructive to a workable, although far from ideal, home-care pattern. The judgment required in situations like this is difficult. St. John's, in practice, has tended to protect the existing care pattern, even if this limits the aggressive rehabilitation of certain respite patients.

Respite Operations

St. John's Home places its two respite beds on a regular SNF unit and tries to assign staff experienced with respite clients to work with respite units. These staff receive in-house training on the special needs of the elderly living at home; the temporary nature of the respite stay and how this temporary stay may involve different care practices to incorporate the patterns of the at-home caregiver; and understanding the caregiver/care recipient unit. As discussed above, the home-visit team is carefully trained to screen potential respite candidates for appropriateness and to refer inappropriate clients to other services. Since the same cadre of nursing home staff usually works with respite, returning clients usually see familiar faces on subsequent visits.

Marketing is critical. St. John's attributes its high occupancy rate to a constant monitoring of reservations, the "back-up" reservation system, and referrals established with other agencies.

RESPITE CARE IN HOSPITALS

Six survey respondents reported offering respite in an acute-care setting. Another four hospital-based programs submitted surveys after the data for this study had been entered on computer and processed. Please note, however, that only the original six are reflected in the survey findings and analysis.

Of the ten programs, six are in Veterans Administration (VA) hospitals, and three are in community acute-care hospitals. HotelHospital, one of the two hospital case studies, is sponsored by an acute-care hospital, but is located in a non-medical care building on its campus and is licensed, surprisingly, as an adult care facility. All VA hospitals offer respite either at little or no cost, but service is limited to veterans. Veterans Administration programs interpret the respite recipient as the elder and not the caregiver, so the service is only available to families when the veteran is the elder receiving respite. The three acute-care programs serve private-pay patients only. HotelHospital services private-pay patients only, but has private funds to underwrite costs for patients who cannot pay.

Benefits to Caregiver and Elders

Hospital respite programs have distinct characteristics, some of which are highly beneficial to caregivers and elders. Others, if not modified, may make this setting inappropriate for some respite users. Because the hospital is intended to serve patients who need a high level of nursing care, it is an ideal place for the elder with multiple and complex medical diagnoses, especially when SNF respite beds are hard to obtain. The availability of medical intervention may soothe some anxious caregivers. At the same time, however, it may make for an unwelcome locale for an elder who is used to a homelike atmosphere.

Some hospitals choose to place the respite unit on their alternate level of care unit (the unit for patients waiting for nursing home placement). This means that clients receive activities and recreation. Others may choose to provide the respite client with special volunteers to provide stimulation.

How individual hospital respite programs develop a homelike atmosphere is not as important as the fact that they are actively working to create one. Consumers would do well to tour the hospital before placing a mentally alert elder there to assure that their elder is treated as a respite client and not as an acute-care patient.

Another concern with hospital-based respite sites is the possibility of nosocomial infections. Existing hospital-based respite programs did not report problems in this area, but the possibility of a frail elder's picking up an infection in an acute-care hospital may be greater than in other settings.

Despite these drawbacks, hospitals can be the respite location of choice for some clients, because the level of medical and nursing care is high. While hospital respite programs generally require that a respite patient be non-acute upon admission, patients needing a great deal of medical supervision can be served with the assurance of on-site medical intervention if needed.

Secondly, some hospitals can take respite patients, if a bed is available, on an emergency basis. Most other programs have pre-admission requirements that preclude emergency placement. Hospital emergency rooms had become a de facto place for relatives under stress to drop off elders in an emergency. A legitimate, planned respite program in a hospital can avert the misuse of the emergency room.

Costs

Of the six hospitals included in the survey, the range of daily fees varied from $55 to $85, with a mean of $66.

Operational Viability

Recent changes in hospital reimbursement have in turn created major changes in hospital bed usage. In many areas, hospitals with underutilized beds can, with appropriate state approval, be assigned to respite. In these hospitals, respite can be seen as both a community service and as a chance for new revenue.

The major challenge faced by hospitals that offer respite lies in recognizing the difference in care needed for respite patients and acute-care patients. The respite client should not be in hospital pajamas nor have regular blood pressure and temperature taken just because such procedures are protocol for all patients. A "respite protocol" to ensure a relatively homelike environment is essential.

Case Study D-1: Respite Care at a VA Medical Center

The Albany, New York VA Medical Center offers hospital-based respite to provide temporary relief for caregivers of chronically ill or disabled veterans. It serves up to six clients at a time in an extended-care wing. It is available only when the recipient is a veteran and only up to 30 days per calendar year. There is no charge for 96 percent of the clients, but in a few cases the Medicare deductible is applied on a sliding scale. The following case study describes only the program at the Albany VA Medical Center.

Program Description

The program uses two private rooms and a four-bed unit in one wing of the extended care unit. Respite stays are for a minimum of one week to a maximum of four weeks. The average length of stay is 11 days. The Albany VA is committed to servicing elderly veterans through this respite program, home health care, adult day care, and caregiver support groups. Respite clients are often recruited from these groups. Respite clients receive the same array of nursing, social, and recreational services available to all patients on that unit.

Recruitment and Admission

A brochure describing the program is distributed widely, and the program is included in the general publicity of an area consortium of geriatric respite services. Referrals are generally made in-house or from other local service agencies.

Using the definition of respite as a service geared toward both caregiver and elder, the VA is in the difficult position of marketing a service that supports only the frail elderly veteran, not the stressed veteran who may be caring for a nonveteran parent or spouse. When veterans in this situation call, they are referred to other local respite services, but otherwise this issue is not specifically addressed.

The admission process is similar to that of St. John's Nursing Home, described earlier. After application forms are completed, the respite coordinator, who is a certified social worker, and an RN either conduct a home visit or visit the prospective client at the VA adult day care program. The visit involves the caregiver, who is informed of the temporary nature of the respite stay. Caregivers who clearly seek permanent nursing home placement are not admitted. A medical "statement of stability" from the family physician is requested. The care plan is reviewed at this time. A signed contract specifying a "release" date reduces delayed discharges.

Because the unit has only two private rooms and the four-bed unit, scheduling becomes a critical part of the admission process. Optimally, a client with dementia should have a private room. Many other clients also prefer private rooms, so the admission process can be slowed because of availability.

The respite coordinator is considering requiring that prospective clients visit the respite unit prior to the stay, both to reduce apprehension and also to give the family seeking respite a realistic view of what can be expected on the extended-care unit, where patients awaiting nursing home placement stay. The environment is unlike HotelHospital, the other hospital-based respite service described in this chapter. The respite experience at the VA has a definite institutional quality. Clients awaiting nursing home placement are often disoriented, and the common rooms are more hospital-like. The atmosphere can be unsettling for a mentally alert respite patient. Advance knowledge of what the situation will be may relieve uneasiness during the stay.

Management and Operations

The respite coordinator is also the social worker in charge of social work services on the extended care unit. This arrangement works well, allowing for close observation of respite patients. The coordinator checks in with each client daily, both for a friendly visit and to assess that support staff is meeting the respite client's needs. For example, have they been taken to appropriate therapies? Are any care problems existing?

A lounge designated only for respite clients allows these clients a separate location to watch TV, meet with other respite clients, or read. Because the VA respite program has an average occupancy rate of 80 percent, it is not uncommon for respite clients to meet and form friendships. That mentally intact respite clients do bond in this manner ameliorates the problem of placing mentally intact elders on a unit with many impaired patients awaiting long-term care placement. Respite patients receive therapies twice a day, usually one session of physical therapy and one of manual arts. The program is self-sufficient at an 80 percent occupancy rate.

In a comprehensive effort to evaluate its own program, the VA conducted a respite-user survey. It found that overall positive experiences were reported by respite clients. Ninety percent stated they would definitely return for another respite visit, and 10 percent responded that they would not use the program again, due mostly to difficulty adjusting to the hospital/nursing home setting.

The survey data supported a change of ward location for the respite care program and increased daily activities for respite patients. Other recommendations were to expand services by using the existing day services program as a day-time respite service, to make arrangements to accommodate patients with severe dementias, and to create a homier environment.

To improve the overall respite census, the VA is developing an on-call list for clients to replace respite patients who cancel reservations at the last minute.

Case Study D-2: Respite Care at a HotelHospital

Presbyterian-University of Pennsylvania Medical Center in Philadelphia
offers a 24-bed unit in a separate building on its hospital campus for
geriatric respite clients, pre- and post-hospital clients, and a vacation suite
("health hotel") for people whose medical conditions make a traditional
hotel unacceptable. The unit offers respite at the personal care level and
has operated successfully for three years.

HotelHospital was chosen for this case study because its integration
of personal care respite with other outpatient temporary care services
demonstrates a unique mode of respite delivery. Since it only offers care
for relatively intact elders, it is distinct from other hospital-based respite
programs that can serve patients needing high levels of care. HotelH-
ospital is the first model nationwide of this type of respite care.

Program Description

The geriatric respite program shares a 24-bed unit with pre- and post-hospital patients, people on vacation, and permanent adult care patients.
Eight to 12 beds are usually used for respite purposes. According to staff,
permanent residents offer a stability to the residents by providing temporary residents with ongoing orientation, reassurance, and companionship.

The goal of the respite stay is to enhance what the staff calls "social
wellness." The unit is licensed as a personal care facility by the Common-
wealth of Pennsylvania. It has a staff of twelve, including LPNs, aides, and
an administrator. Volunteers supplement care. The daily rate is $60 for a
semi-private, $75 for a private room.

Recruitment and Admission

Although a series of attractive brochures on outpatient services was widely
distributed, staff felt strongly that "word of mouth" was clearly the best
method of recruitment. As with other successful respite programs, many
respite clients repeat their stay at HotelHospital. Several post-service
procedures provide ongoing contact, which would seem to encourage
repeat stays. These procedures include both telephone and written fol-
low-ups, a post-stay evaluation, and birthday cards. Staff reports that
post-stay communication is two-way: Respite clients occasionally call to
keep in contact with respite staff. Word-of-mouth referrals are abetted by
supplying former respite clients with a series of brochures to give to
friends.

The admission process for respite usually involves a visit to the hospital unit by the elder, a required report by the elder's physician, a conference with both caregiver and client, a facility tour, and the development of an emergency and a discharge plan.Since the unit is licensed at the board-and-care level, not all elders living in the community are appropriate for respite. Only patients who are independent in activities of daily living (ADLs) and who have a minimum of mental impairments are suitable. Some heavy care respite candidates, however, are admitted occasionally if the projected census at the time of the stay shows most clients to be at a light level of care, thus freeing staff to care adequately for the respite client. An occasional client is admitted on an emergency basis from the hospital's emergency room. Respite staff assesses such clients in the emergency room to assure that they can be served by the respite program. The two respite beds are filled at a rate of approximately 80 percent. A private grant can cover immediate costs of an emergency placement of clients who are unable to pay full fees.

Respite Operations

HotelHospital is extremely cheerful. Upon entering, the visitor sees snapshots of former and present clients and staff. TVs, board games, and cards are being fully utilized in a large multipurpose dining and activity room.

Respite clients are urged, but not forced, to join the social environment. Clients whose respite was longer limits of the respite stay (the minimum is three days; the maximum is three weeks) are encouraged to help orient and welcome newer temporary visitors. The cheerful, informal ambiance of the unit seems to result in a "pride of place" that is evident in both residents and staff. Some clients frequently repeat three-day weekends.

The personality and professionalism of staff is clearly the agent creating this ambiance. Staff is permanently assigned and specially selected for this unit. Staff training is done individually by the administrator. The content of training is geared toward making the patient feel useful and wanted, but it includes an overview of what "respite" entails in terms of both elder and caregiver.

Services to caregivers are informal. Staff helps caregivers forge linkages to appropriate community services and support groups. Changes in the health or mental status of the respite recipient are fully discussed. Positive changes are often explained to caregivers using the experience within the unit of feeling part of a group and feeling useful.

COMBINATION MODELS

Twenty-three percent of respondents reported that they offer more than one kind of respite service. Typical combinations were institutional/adult home and institutional/home-based. The case study of the Metropolitan Commission on Aging of Syracuse, New York provides details on a program of this kind.

Benefits and Drawbacks to Consumers

There are no major changes in the benefits and drawbacks of a respite service when it is offered in conjunction with another model of respite. An additional plus, however, may result from the potential of choice. In this model, one telephone call can alert a caregiver to respite options. In independent programs, several calls to different agencies may be needed to find out what respite services are available. The respite coordinator in a combined program may also be able to help clients choose the respite service that meets their needs best.

Costs

All combined programs reported cases separately for each program.

Operational Viability

The major operational benefit of a combined program is that it can offer prospective clients an alternative if one mode of service is unavailable. Otherwise, the strengths and weaknesses of each model remain.

Case Study E: Respite Care from Home Aides

This respite program operates under a direct provision-of-service model. A full-time respite coordinator matches the needs of respite clients with the availability of care that is provided either in the home or an institution. The program has a sliding fee schedule, using funds allocated by the New York State legislature and managed by the New York State Department of Social Services. This sliding scale mechanism, unique to Syracuse, is called "fiscal access."

Program Description

A respite coordinator, employed by Home Aides of Central New York, administers the program and reports to the executive director of that agency. The Metropolitan Commission on Aging, the agency that actually receives respite funds for management and fee subsidies from the State of New York, subcontracts with the home aides for the provision of respite care. The program receives additional guidance from a Respite Advisory Committee. Several agencies participate in this respite care program. Home Aides of Central New York employs not only the respite coordinator but also the home care paraprofessionals who provide the in-home care. Plaza Health and Rehabilitation Center provides most of the skilled care, while James Square Nursing Home and St. Camillus Health and Rehabilitation Center provide ICF and additional SNF institutional care. Bellevue Manor provides adult care in its residence. The skilled nursing facilities do not reserve beds for respite clients, according to the respite coordinator; however, respite clients can almost always be accommodated in one of these institutions. If an emergency necessitates immediate in-home service, Home Aides of Central New York is equipped to provide service immediately. The average length of stay for all services is 10 days.

Recruitment and Admission

This program, like only 31 percent of programs in our survey, can admit clients regardless of their ability to pay or their eligibility for Medicaid. General marketing, therefore, is appropriate. The respite coordinator reports that the service is best marketed through paid advertising in small community newspapers, followed by radio spots, public presentations and by maintaining close contact with other agencies that serve the aged.

Despite five years of active marketing of the service, new clients are often surprised and pleased to learn of the program, according to the respite staff. This fact reinforces the need to develop marketing strategies for people independent of the traditional aging services delivery system.

The respite coordinator conducts an initial telephone assessment of all new cases and provides information and referral to other agencies when the client is inappropriate or ineligible for respite care. In appropriate situations, the respite coordinator and the agency community health nurse conduct a home assessment. This assessment includes a PRI (patient review instrument) and a related screen used in New York State to determine both the level and the setting of care. In this program, the PRI serves as a reference point for determining which level of in-home services will be best. The home visit is also used to emphasize the temporary nature of respite care, to reach agreement with the caregiver concerning the proposed care plan recommended by the coordinator and nurse and to establish a firm discharge date and discharge plan.

Once the required service is agreed upon by the coordinator, nurse, and family, the coordinator makes arrangements with the appropriate agency for the exact dates and helps the family work through the admission procedures. Eligibility for the sliding scale subsidy is also discussed during the home visit, and a payment rate is negotiated. Subsidies are based upon monthly income and expenses.

Operations

Each participating agency follows its own operational protocols for respite, similar in some ways to the operational details of the St. John's and INTERAC models. The variety of choices of care settings the caregiver has is the most obvious benefit of this model. With one telephone call and one home visit, the coordinator can arrange for the service to begin. The coordinator reports that some families initially resist institutional placements, although over a 5-year period, institutional placement (338 respite stays) has been slightly more common than in-home respite (293 respite services). These statistics become even more interesting, since the nursing home does not set aside beds for respite. This indicates that, at least in some cases, clients could not be served institutionally.

When home care is chosen, the PRI assessment helps determine which level of care, companion-homemaker or home health aide, is more appropriate. The home care worker often provides assistance on a "live-in" basis, sometimes for the duration of the respite service. In the case of dementia clients, home health aides are assigned to 12-hour shifts to ensure continuity of care. Home health aides are also used when significant medical problems exist. In this program, no home care workers are hired to provide exclusive respite services. All home health aides who serve respite clients have successfully completed a New York State-approved training program at Home Aides of Central New York.

Companion-homemakers used on respite cases are employed by a subsidiary of Home Aides of Central New York. In each instance, workers receive the same pay as they would if they were on regular cases of the agency. The actual respite fee is based upon the families' ability to pay.

When institutional care is the choice for respite service, participants follow the full admission procedure of the facility that provides the care. Admission agreements are discussed with the family and signed at the time of admission. This agreement not only provides for admission, but also ensures that all parties agree to the date and time of discharge. In its five-year report, Home Aides of Central New York indicates that out of 338 institutional placements, 299 were at the SNF level, 16 at the ICF level, and 23 at the adult home level.

The respite coordinator has established quality assurance mechanisms. The respite coordinator maintains daily telephone contact with the worker on all in-home cases and uses the results of post-stay evaluations as an additional method of quality assurance. In cases of both in-home and institutional respite care, service is regulated by quality assurance protocols of the agency providing care.

REFERENCES

Perdue, J. Respite care for the frail or disabled elderly. *Pride Inst. J. Long-Term Home Health Care* 3(4):81-87, 1984.

Scharlach, A. and C. Prenzel. Evaluation of institution-based respite care. *Gerontologist* 26(1):77-82, 1986.

SUGGESTED READINGS

Bader, J. Respite care: temporary relief for caregivers. *Women and Health* 10(2-3):39-52, 1985.

Brown County Respite Care. *A Training Manual for Respite Care Providers.* Green Bay, WI: Brown County Respite Care, 1988.

California Program Serves Families of Brain-Damaged Adults. *Aging* 341:30-35, 1988.

Crossman, L., C. London and C. Barry. Older women caring for disabled spouses: a model for supportive services. *Gerontologist* 21(5): 1981.

Crozier, M.C. Respite care keeps elders at home longer. *Perspectives on Aging* 11(5): 1982.

Dunn, R. et al. Respite admissions and the disabled elderly. *Am. Geriatrics Soc. J.* 81(10):613-616, 1988.

Ellis, V. and D. Wilson. A model respite program. *Clin. Gerontol.* 1(1):100-101:1982.

Foundation for Long-Term Care. *Respite Care for the Frail Elderly: A Summary Report on Institutional Respite Research and Operation Manual.* Albany, NY: The Center for the Study of Aging, 1983.

Hasselkus, B. and M. Brown. Respite care for community elderly. *Am. J. Occup. Ther.* 37(2):83-88, 1983.

Hildebrant, E., et al. Respite care. *Am. J. Nursing* 83(10):1428-1434, 1983.

Lidoff, L. *Respite Companion Program Model.* Washington, DC: The National Council on the Aging, 1983.

Loss, I. *Elder Care Share Manual.* Kalamazoo, MI: Southcentral Michigan Commission on Aging, 1985.

Meltzer, J. *Respite Care: An Emerging Family Support Service.* Washington, DC: The Center for the Study of Social Policy, 1982.

Netting, F.E. and L.N. Kennedy. Project RENEW: development of a volunteer respite care program. *Gerontologist* 25(6):578-576, 1985.

Newald, J. Women as caregivers face crisis at home. *Hospital* 6(60):106, 1986.

New York State Department of Social Services. *Respite Demonstration Project.* Albany, NY: New York State Department of Social Services, 1986.

Older Women's League. *Respite Services for Caregivers: A Model State Bill.* Washington, DC: Older Women's League, 1987.

Project SHARE. Respite and Crisis Care. Human Services Bibliography Series. Rockville, MD: Project SHARE, 1981.

Project SHARE. *How-to Manual on Providing Respite Care for Family Caregivers.* Rockville, MD: Project SHARE, 1985.

Sands, D. and T. Suzuki. Adult day care for Alzheimer's patients and their families. Gerontologist 28(1):21-28, 1988.

Schwartz, S. and R. Dobrof. In T. Quinn and J. Crabtree, eds., *How to Start a Respite Service for People with Alzheimer's and Their Families.* New York: The Brookdale Foundation and the Brookdale Center on Aging of Hunter College, 1987.

Spence, D.L. and D.B. Miller. Family respite for the elderly Alzheimer's patient. *J. Geront. Social Work* 9(2):101-112, 1985.

Stone, R. *Recent Developments in Respite Care Services for Caregivers of the Frail Elderly.* San Francisco: Aging Health Policy Center, University of California, 1985.

Warren, R. and I.R. Dickman. For This Respite, Much Thanks. In *Concepts, Guidelines and Issues in the Development of Community Respite Care Services for Families of Persons with Developmental Disabilities.* New York: United Cerebral Palsy Associations, Inc., 1981.

Yocum, B. *Respite Care Options for Families Caring for the Frail Elderly* Seattle: University of Washington, Pacific Northwest Long-Term Care Center, 1982.

2

Innovative Institutional
Approaches to Respite Care

Theresa L. Martico-Greenfield, MPH

The Jewish Home and Hospital for Aged (JHHA), the teaching nursing home affiliate of Mount Sinai Medical Center, has numerous programs that serve more than 3000 well and frail elderly. Among these programs are three long-term care facilities (1600 beds) as well as three senior housing environments (Enriched Housing, Kaufmann Residence and Kittay House). In addition, The Jewish Home has a Short-Stay Inpatient Rehabilitation Unit, Adult Day Care (for frail elderly, individuals with Alzheimer's and other dementias and for the visually impaired elderly), Long-Term Home Health Care, Geriatric Outreach and Alzheimer's In-Home Emergency Respite.

Unlike many other nursing homes, JHHA does not formally provide institution-based respite care—for regulatory and financial, as well as logistical reasons. In addition, reimbursement rates and regulatory requirements for assessment, care planning and discharge planning were revised in 1991. Space configuration and bed availability are other factors that precluded the offering of this service. Instead, The Home has viewed its community programs as the primary resource for respite services.

The Alzheimer's In-Home Emergency Respite Program is the only program offered at JHHA that was established as a formal respite service. The following case examples illustrate the reasons this service was needed:

Joan takes care of her father who suffers from Alzheimer's disease. Joan would like the opportunity to visit her daughter for a few days on the West

Coast to meet her new granddaughter. She cannot, however, find anyone who will take care of her father for more than a few hours at a time.

Herb needs to take a few days off for a minor surgical procedure. However, he cannot find the professional help needed to care for his mother who has Alzheimer's disease. Herb feels there is no one he can turn to who will understand his mother's erratic behavior and how to cope with her in his absence.

Marge and Fred have taken care of Fred's grandmother who has suffered from Alzheimer's disease for a number of years. Marge says she is "about to climb the wall," and she and Fred long to get away for just a few days by themselves. They are despondent because they do not know how to find someone sufficiently trained to handle his grandmother's agitation and severe memory loss.

Established in 1987 with a generous grant from Mutual of New York (MONY) Financial Services, the Alzheimer's Disease In-Home Emergency Respite Program ensures the continuity of home care in familiar and comfortable surroundings for individuals with Alzheimer's disease and at the same time permits family members a 3- to 7-day period in which they can attend to personal matters. Before the service is implemented, a registered nurse and a social worker visit the family to evaluate the individual and to learn his daily routine.

Home health aides for this program must have excellent work experience and training in the field. In addition, they must successfully complete a 25-hour, intensive training course in the care of Alzheimer's patients taught by JHHA staff. To further ensure the quality of the program, JHHA's nurses observe and monitor the work of the aides in the home environment and are available for consultation at all times. The program also features family counseling and linkage to other Alzheimer's disease services. The major benefits of the program for the caregiver and individual with Alzheimer's disease are:

- It responds to the need for professional respite care for Alzheimer's patients and their families.
- It provides peace of mind to caregivers who will no longer be forced to rely on makeshift services when emergencies demand separation from their impaired relatives.
- It provides respite in the individual's own home instead of in a temporary institution. This avoids increased stress, anxiety, confusion and agitation, to which individuals with Alzheimer's disease are particularly vulnerable.
- It provides a tailor-made program that address the individual needs

of each person. The home care staff learns the daily routine and the likes and dislikes of each individual before providing services.

In the spring of 1988 we trained ten home health aides who were selected from the dozens of home health aides known to The Home's Long-Term Home Health Care programs. The home health aides who provide the direct respite service were required to complete a 25-hour curriculum—the Alzheimer's Respite Care Training Program (ARCTP)—a 3-day intensive training program. The program teaches home health aides how to provide safe, quality care to Alzheimer's patients in their homes in the absence of their families. The training program combines theory and practice through group discussion, individual participation, and role playing. On the first day of training participants are asked to complete a Pre-Program Self-Evaluation form and to keep it until the last day of training. On the last day of training the participant is asked to complete a Post-Program Self-Evaluation form. The instructor then gives the correct responses to the questions on the evaluation form and asks the participant to compare the number of correct responses on the pre-evaluation form to the number of correct responses on the post-evaluation form. Since the pre- and post-evaluation form is the same, it allows for the evaluation of baseline knowledge and individual learning. A certificate is presented to the participants upon successful completion of the program.

The curriculum topics were as follows:

1. What is Alzheimer's Disease?
2. Through New Eyes: Changes in Perception due to Alzheimer's Disease
3. Understanding the Relationship Between Personality and Behavior in Caring for the Dementia Patient
4. Breaking the Code: Communicating with People with Alzheimer's Disease
5. Patient Safety and Accident Prevention
6. The World Turned Upside Down: Behavioral Changes in People with Alzheimer's Disease
7. Family Relationships and Concerns: How They are Influenced by the Behavior of Patients with Alzheimer's Disease
8. Medical/Nursing Interventions Utilized with Alzheimer's Patients
9. Nutrition and Elimination Needs of Alzheimer's Patients
10. People with Alzheimer's Disease and Their Families: I Don't Know You Anymore
11. Activity and Rest Needs of Alzheimer's Patients

12. Getting Help: How and When

The plan for respite service begins with a telephone inquiry and interview by the program director who is a registered nurse with many years' experience in home care. Once it is determined that respite services are needed, an appointment is made for a home assessment by a registered nurse and social worker to determine the amount of physical care the individual will require and the type of behavioral and emotional issues that may arise. In this way the most appropriate match between the specially trained home health aides and the older person can be achieved. Once the service plan is developed and has started, a registered nurse monitors and supervises the home health aide.

In the 4 years since the program's inception almost 300 inquiries have been received, resulting in service to 40 families. Most inquiries were from caregivers—spouses and adult children—who were planning for future needs. (These calls were handled primarily by a social worker and lasted from 20 to 45 minutes each.)

Almost from the start of the program variations on the 24-hour-per-day service have been provided, with most families using between 8 and 12 hours per day of service for up to 7 consecutive days. The service has been used by caregivers who had medical care needs themselves, such as unexpected hospitalizations or elective surgery; who had vacations or who had to travel to be with other family members.

During the 4 years that this service has been offered, many useful and important lessons have been learned. Initially, the Home's outreach efforts focused largely on the needs of caregivers for this service, thereby identifying caregivers as the client. Experience and research has demonstrated that family caregivers cannot—or will not—identify themselves as the party in need of service; perhaps it causes feelings of inadequacy or the belief that they have failed in their role as caregivers. As a result, the outreach has shifted it's focus to how this service meets the needs of the individual with Alzheimer's disease differently, or better than, other available alternatives.

We also learned that caregivers often use informal networks made up of family members and friends when they have to go away for long periods of time. This is often because they feel anxious and unsure about having a "stranger" staying in their relative's home while they are away. Caregivers seemed to be more interested in having an in-home respite service available for several hours a day, a few days each week (as opposed to more time) so that they could either work part-time, address their own children's needs, or take care of other personal matters. We then had to look at the structure of the program and consider whether the in-depth nursing and social work assessments that we were providing were necessary for this type of respite service. The nursing assessment appeared to be more critical to a successful plan of care, and the social work assessment could be made as the nurse deemed necessary.

Financially, this service is expensive to provide and even more expensive for family caregivers to afford, primarily because neither Medicare nor Medicaid pays for such a service. A sliding fee scale was developed with a minimum rate of $30 per day up to the full rate (that is, the full cost) of $275 per day. The grant from MONY Financial Services is dedicated to providing subsidies to the caregivers, but it is often difficult to determine how much the caregiver can afford to contribute toward the cost. The issue of whether only the older persons' financial circumstances should be considered (as opposed to the family caregiver) in making this determination; after all, the services were being provided directly to them.

Other general impressions have been that (1) caregivers will often wait until the point of crisis to seek help; (2) caregivers need a lot of support prior to accepting services (for example, up to 90 minutes of telephone contact is usually provided by the social worker in the weeks leading up to the time services are needed); (3) long-term counseling is often indicated but generally not sought by caregivers. The response to the service once it has been provided has been highly gratifying; caregivers have expressed great appreciation for the service and most feel that it has helped a great deal.

The second type of community-based respite offered by JHHA is geriatric day care, now in three different settings. Now 18 years old, the geriatric day center at the Bronx Division was the first program of this sort established in a nursing home. It is a medical model program, reimbursable by Medicaid and serves 200 members in total. Day center members arrive at 9:00 a.m. and stay until 3:00 p.m., 7 days a week. Transportation service is provided by The Home. Each program day is filled with therapeutic recreation programs, rehabilitation services, nursing consultations, social work services and opportunities for socializing with new and old friends. A hot lunch is provided as is an afternoon snack. Members typically come to the program two or three times a week.

The day center program was replicated in collaboration with the Jewish Guild for the Blind for older individuals with visual impairments and takes place at The Home as well. Specially trained staff work with the members in this program, which services 60 in total.

The geriatric day center at the Manhattan Division has grown dramatically in its 4 years of operation. It is also a 7-day-a-week, medical model program that serves up to 200 clients.

Many day center members have mild dementia. Programming is

developed both in an integrated fashion as well as separately where only members with dementia will take part. This is done so that members can select and be assisted in selecting activities that minimize frustration, maximize self-esteem and provide enjoyment during the day.

These programs are an excellent resource for caregivers because they encompass the entire day and are available on weekends. Often, the geriatric day center programs are the difference between a caregiver being able to continue working or not. The program also offers medical and nursing support which can prevent serious problems from arising. In some instances, when coupled with home care services, the geriatric day center can enable an elderly individual to remain in the community rather than having to enter a nursing facility.

The Jewish Home also offers long-term home health care through the "Nursing Home Without Walls" program to approximately 600 individuals in Manhattan and the Bronx. Primarily a Medicaid-funded program, long-term home health care is designed to provide the same level of nursing care for individuals that they would receive in a nursing facility, but at 75 percent of the cost. Rehabilitation, nutrition, social work and transportation services as needed are also part of the care plan. Unlike day care this program addresses the needs of the homebound individual. One of the requirements for this program is that someone—either the client or a caregiver—direct and supervise the home care services. Thus, while caregivers must often be available, they can continue to work, raise a family and maintain their lifestyle with the help of the long-term home health care program.

A particular benefit to caregivers from all of these services is the support provided by the social service component. Counseling is available at all times so that the caregiver is not alone in considering different treatment alternatives, placement in a nursing home, financial options, or entitlements. The value of a long-term relationship with a particular program or facility cannot be overestimated, especially as decision-making points arise.

In general, we have found that transitions between programs and levels of care occur with less anxiety and more confidence because the element of the "unknown quantity" is almost eliminated. In addition, program staff will remain involved through the initial adjustment—for example, from day care to nursing home placement—so that the nursing home can benefit from their knowledge of the individual and his family.

The JHHA's approach to respite strives to provide the greatest benefit for the individual, the caregiver, the community and the health care system while recognizing that the individual's quality of life is the most significant consideration of all.

3

Inpatient Respite in the Provision of Palliative Care

Terry Kinzel, MD

Palliative or hospice care is increasingly recognized as a valid adjunct to traditional medical care of the terminally ill cancer patient. The concept of respite care as temporary relief for the caregiver was developed primarily for families of patients with dementia, however this concept can also serve as a valuable component of a comprehensive palliative care program. The benefits of inpatient hospital respite care for terminally ill patients include improved diagnosis and therefore improved symptom control, the opportunity to intensify symptom control in a safer setting, intensive caregiver training and the opportunity to provide counseling, planning and reassurance in a secure setting while giving the caregivers a breather. Potential problems with inpatient respite include raising the patient's fear of abandonment, some unavoidable aspects of institutional care, and the risk of confusing the goals of care when terminally ill patients are mingled with other patients, such as those in active rehabilitation programs.

PALLIATIVE CARE

Studies show that cancer, accounting for 22 percent of all deaths in 1985 (461,563 compared to 278,562 in 1962), is second only to heart disease as the leading cause of mortality in the United States today. Although there have been significant advances in the diagnosis and treatment of cancer, some forms of cancer may now be cured through early diagnosis, but the most common cancers (lung, prostate, colon/rectum, breast, uterus and ovary) are rarely curable. Even though the 5-year survival rate has increased for several types of cancer, far too many people who develop cancer will eventually die of the disease despite all the therapies modern medicine has to offer. It is for those in the final stages of their illness that the hospice movement was developed.

Hospice care is a physician-directed, nurse-coordinated, interdisciplinary team approach to the care of the terminally ill, available 24 hours a day, 7 days a week. It emphasizes caring treatment of the spiritual and psychological as well as the physical needs of the patient, rather than further attempts at aggressive curative treatment at a point when such treatment has become futile. With palliative care, the goal is to help the patient live as fully and comfortably as possible during the time that remains.

As palliative care reflects a philosophy rather than a structure, several forms have developed: community-based, freestanding, hospital-based team and hospital-based unit. In the United States, the community-based form is most common. This chapter explores how a hospital-based respite program can serve to complement and support community-based hospice.

RESPITE CARE

Respite care developed largely in response to the great numbers of people with dementia and consequently the great number being cared for in the homes of busy families. Like palliative care, respite care has taken several forms: in-home, adult day care and inpatient (usually as a program in a long-term care facility). The primary goal of respite is to provide time and physical and emotional relief to the primary caregiver in order to extend the time the patient can be cared for in the home.

A REPRESENTATIVE FACILITY

Our inpatient program is based in the VA Medical Center, Iron Mountain, Michigan. The medical center is a secondary care hospital in the rural upper peninsula of Michigan with 180 acute care beds, 20 intermediate care beds and 40 Nursing Home Care Unit (NHCU) beds. The Palliative Care Program uses two acute beds and a flexible number of beds on the NHCU, usually averaging about 10. In addition to the regular nursing staff on the units, care is provided by a palliative care team composed of a registered nurse who has additional training in oncology and hospice care, a social worker and a pastor. In addition, the hospital's medical oncologist is actively involved in the palliative care on the acute service. The Geriatrician Director of the NHCU is Director of the Palliative Care Program and responsible for the direct care of the patients in the palliative beds on the NHCU. There is an outreach program for patients in the Medical Oncology Clinic. However, because of the very low population density (with some patients coming from over 250 miles away), direct hospice care in the home is provided by community hospice programs where available. The NHCU has had an active respite care program for over 8 years.

USES OF INPATIENT HOSPICE

In the terminally ill patient, inpatient respite may be useful in a number of ways:

- Diagnosis. As the primary principle of hospice care is to focus on relieving the patient's symptoms, invasive or extensive diagnostic procedures are avoided when possible. However, at times, determining the specific etiology of a symptom is important to effectively treat the symptom. For example, ruling out hypercalcemia as the cause of lethargy, determining the role of congestive heart failure in contributing to dyspnea, or deciding whether dysuria is due to a urinary tract infection. Determinations of this kind can usually be done without invasive procedures and may have a significant impact in the specific treatment aimed at relieving symptoms. Since the workup may involve x-rays or sequential testing, having a patient in a setting where this may be accomplished with a minimum of travel is very helpful.
- Symptom Control. In addition to having an accurate diagnosis of the cause of symptoms, it is frequently easier to gain rapid control of symptoms in an inpatient setting. For instance, if a patient with bony metastasis is having increased pain, the closer observation available in an inpatient respite program allows for a prompt increase in morphine and better observation of the effect of adjunctive therapy such as nonsteroidal anti-inflammatory drugs or steroids. Also, nursing interventions may be carried out more thoroughly and rapidly in a respite program.
- Training. Particularly with nursing interventions such as skin care, bowel programs, administration and monitoring of medications, injections and also areas such as diet evaluation and preparation, intensive training available in an inpatient respite program can better prepare the patient and caregivers to return home.

- Counseling, Planning and Reassurance. A 2-week respite from home care can allow the patient and caregivers to step back from the stress of home care, get advice on how to solve problems and make plans for changes at home. For example, is a hospital bed now necessary? Is additional in-home nursing care necessary?
- Physician Availability. Hospice emphasizes all aspects of care and not just biomedical interventions. However, in many cases optimum relief of symptoms such as pain requires active physician involvement. However, physicians are not readily available in some areas. For example, in the areas served by our program, the community-based hospice programs (located in small, very rural communities, many miles from our center) are voluntary with minimal physician input. The presence of a physician in an inpatient respite program can add greatly to a community program.

PROBLEMS OF INPATIENT RESPITE CARE FOR THE TERMINALLY ILL

While a respite program may be a valuable supplement to home hospice care, several potential problems are inherent in its use.

1. Fear of Abandonment. Although ideally the program will be used for the purposes just described, patients may view the move to an inpatient program as a prelude to abandonment by the family.
2. Institutional Care. When the respite program is housed within an institution, no matter how dedicated and skilled the staff, the care will, by definition, be institutional. The food won't be the same as at home; private rooms are rare; the walls and views are not the same; and even a dedicated nurse isn't the same as a wife of many years.
3. Confusion.
    a. Confusion on the patient's part. For patients with fairly advanced disease, especially if there is any cognitive impairment, moving to a strange place with different schedules and routines may cause disorientation. This is commonly seen in respite programs with dementia patients and although less common in the terminally ill, it may still occur.
    b. Confusion on the staff's part. In good programs, confusion will be minimal, but in a respite program for the terminally ill housed in a multipurpose setting (for example, in a long-term care setting that also serves rehabilitation patients) it requires very clear thinking to keep general goals for palliative patients

separate from the overall goals of the unit. There is a risk of both overtreating and undertreating the patient. Overtreatment comes in the form of performing diagnostic evaluations and therapeutic interventions appropriate for patients without terminal illness who have a relatively long life expectancy. For example, in a patient receiving rehabilitation for an amputation due to peripheral vascular disease, aggressive management of hypertension even at the expense of drug side effects might be warranted; but most likely treatment of hypertension would not be undertaken in someone with extensively metastatic lung cancer. In contrast, the approach to using narcotics in that amputee would be much different than in the terminally ill cancer patient.

CONCLUSION

Hospice care is about life, the life that a patient with a terminal illness has yet to live. The goal of this care is to allow that person to live that life as fully and comfortably as possible. Many techniques have been developed to achieve this goal. Inpatient respite for the terminally ill patient can be a valuable component of a comprehensive program.

4

The Role of a City Office for the Aging in Accessing Respite Services for Caregivers

Sally Robinson, DSW

The following critique of respite care is based upon almost 20 years of experience in a municipal Office for the Aging whose mission includes the delivery and promotion of community resources that enable and support elderly people's ability to manage at home. Central to the ability of older people with functional disabilities to remain in their homes and avoid institutional long-term care is the care they receive from their families. Family caregivers have always been the primary providers of home care to the elderly. Even for a burgeoning population of persons in their eighties and nineties, families continue to be their major caregiving resource. It is generally accepted that relatives provide over 80 percent of all the home care delivered to older adults.

In this services environment, the access of families to practical help in support of their caregiving role is paramount to the mission of Offices for the Aging and other formal public and private providers of long-term community care to the elderly. The effectiveness of any access service is highly associated with the expressed agreement between provider and client as to what is being accessed.

Workers and clients may proceed at cross purposes unless there is clear communication between them regarding the services needed and available. Such an assessment and need vis-à-vis resources to meet that need is most important in relation to respite services for family caregivers.

"Respite from what" should be clearly and fully articulated before services are accessed.

RESPITE AS "TIME OUT"

Typically, respite care is conceptualized and designed as care provided to an elder in the absence of his or her regular caregiver— care that is provided on a replacement basis for the purpose of freeing the natural caregiver from his or her caregiving responsibilities for a specific period of time. Type, scope and duration of these services may vary widely—from a few hours of companionship once a week to a weekend or longer period with overnight supervision which may include extensive personal care. The skills required of on-line providers of respite services vary accordingly. For example, friendly visitor-type respite services may be provided by a volunteer, whereas staff of a community respite center require professional credentials. The elderly with Alzheimer's disease may require a more highly trained respite caregiver than the older person whose frailty does not involve dementia or some other incapacitating mental or physical condition like incontinence.

THE REINVENTION OF RESPITE CARE

The widespread provision of care by families and other informal caregivers has led to a growing realization among formal service providers that services provided under the respite rubric may not be adequately responsive to the needs of natural caregivers unless these services are part of an integrated caregiver support plan. Respite care has to be reinvented in order to assure that respite opportunities are evaluated and accessed as response to one type of caregiving need rather than as the sole—or primary—support need of natural caregivers.

Practice experience has revealed that respite care is more or less accessible and maximized by the availability of those case planning and management services that include their assessment of caregiver ability and willingness to provide care. Adult children or other family members who provide care for their elderly relatives only because other resources appear to be unavailable require more respite services. These caregivers need assistance in accessing primary caregiving alternatives. The association between unwillingness to provide care and elder abuse is observed, especially when the caregiver's unwillingness is complicated by unreasonable demands from care recipients. Social workers and other professionals involved in care planning with older people and their families must be alert to evidence of reluctance of family members to meet some or all of the care needs of their elderly relatives. Assessment must determine caregiver willingness. Too often, based perhaps on strongly held family values of obligation and reciprocity between generations, families find it difficult to accept in themselves or to let others know of their unwillingness to provide primary care, or at least certain types of care. For the same reasons, professionals may presume a willingness of family members to provide primary care, and then later they may blame the limited availability of respite services as the major factor in a dysfunctional or abusive caregiving situation. Both the elder's care needs and the family caregiver's willingness must be analyzed in terms of tasks.

Ability to provide care is also a major factor in family caregiving. A willingness to provide care is not enough, especially when that willingness is mainly the result of feelings of obligation and responsibility that people typically feel for their relatives. Caregiver burden should not be linked to need for respite services unless and until the caregiver's financial, physical, intellectual and emotional ability to provide care is assessed and addressed. This step in accessing respite services is crucial. A willing caregiver may deny inability. Caregivers who are burdened by an inability to meet what may be unrealistic caregiving demands and standards may reject respite opportunities. They may feel guilty about leaving the care recipient, or they may feel that their caregiving inadequacies will be observed by the respite provider. The complexity of individual family characteristics and dynamics requires a use of respite services that takes into account the impact of these characteristics and dynamics on the caregiving situation in general and on the value of respite services in particular.

A PROTOCOL FOR THE ASSESSMENT OF RESPITE AND OTHER COMMUNITY SUPPORT NEEDS AND CAPABILITIES OF FAMILY CAREGIVERS

Since family caregiving responsibilities may begin or change with the hospitalization of an elderly relative, thorough assessment or reassessment of informal caregiving capability should be done when an elderly patient's discharge plan includes primary caregiving by a family member. The charts of these patients should be flagged for a followup with their family caregivers by appropriate hospital discharge planning personnel or by social workers from the local Office for the Aging or other community social care agency. The patients and their physicians should contribute to the caregiving assessment process in order to assure that the patient's medical needs and regimen can be adequately supported by family caregivers. The family's willingness and ability in this regard should be examined, ideally, with the consensus of all concerned as to whether the family can handle primary caregiving responsibility. If it is determined that the family's role can be primary, the need for supplemental formal support can then be assessed. The role of the Office for the Aging or other community service agency in assessing formal support services, including respite opportunities, is only applicable after the parameters of family and other informal caregiving are realistically determined and agreed upon. Only when coordinated, systematic planning has been done can respite services be properly assessed and put into place. The application of respite services to a family caregiving situation alone does not assure the success of that situation unless respite is delivered as part of an individuated, integrated community support system. As such, respite services may mainly be an intermission in family caregiving responsibilities, or other services that reduce caregiver burden. For example, services such as peer support groups, training in caregiving techniques and psychosocial counseling may free family caregivers from psychological or physical stress in that these services can strengthen the ability of caregivers to meet their caregiving responsibilities. As well, a maximized ability to provide care may promote a family caregiver's willingness to initiate or sustain care.

THE RESPITE USE OF COMMUNITY SUPPORT SERVICES FOR THE ELDERLY

Although the array of services available under the Older American's Act and other federal and state legislation was not designed to meet the respite needs of family caregivers, many are, in fact, used for this purpose. These services include both medical and social day care, congregate and home-delivered meals, transportation assistance, advice about entitlements—including assistance in the negotiation of bureaucracies like public welfare institutions and Social Security—case management services that include social needs assessment and the assessing of social care resources and age-specific recreational resources. Publicly subsidized home care resources also are sought by family caregivers as respite services. That is, families may seek support of their caregiving rather than the supplantation of their efforts by formal alternatives, alternatives to which their elderly relative may have a statutory entitlement.

SPECIAL RESPITE NEEDS OF CAREGIVING SPOUSES OF ALZHEIMER'S PATIENTS

Office for the Aging case management services are increasingly directed to the needs of elderly patients with Alzheimer's disease and their caregiving spouses. These natural caregiving situations may place the caregiver at special social, psychological and personal health risk due to the heightened and agitated anxiety that often afflicts the care recipient suffering from Alzheimer's disease. Many of these patients demand the constant presence and attention of their caregiving spouse or relatives. The persistent anxiety of these patients may also keep them and their spouses awake most of the night. Without respite, the caregiving spouses and relatives, many of whom—to complicate matters—have their own health problems, cannot sustain their caregiving. The result of these situations? The primary caregiver may become acutely ill and require hospitalization. Or, out of desperation, and a perceived lack of alternatives makes the institutionalization of the Alzheimer's patient as the only alternative. With the assistance of respite services, the caregiving spouse may be able to continue their caregiving throughout the course of their spouse's illness. When these caregiving situations can be maintained without major changes and undue burden to the caregivers, both care recipients and their caregivers benefit. Regularly scheduled discussions that concentrate on the responsibilities of the caregiver can make all the difference in these situations, especially when the separation anxiety of the care recipient is addressed. The provision of respite care in the same facility and at the same time of respite care in a group setting and of caregiver training, also in a group, can be effective in this regard. The care recipient is reassured by the close proximity of the caregiver; and the caregivers are similarly at ease because they know that they are available to their spouse when needed. Both care recipient and caregiver receive the attention and support of concerned others. In such programs, the caregiver's peer support group can follow training so that a weekly intermission can be continued for both care recipient and caregiver.

CONCLUSION

This chapter has introduced several key aspects of the role of an Office for the Aging in the access to respite services of family caregivers of the elderly. As a pivotal organization in the development and delivery of community-based long-term care, it is incumbent upon municipal Offices on Aging to assure a managed approach to the access of respite services so that these opportunities are relevant and effective components in an integrated, comprehensive supportive care system.

5

Adult Day Care as an Alternative to Long-Term Institutionalization for the Frail Elderly

Tamara Robin Jasper, MSW

Ten years ago in June, my father started acting funny. He and my mother had just driven up from Florida to spend the summer at their country home in northern Westchester County. When I came to visit them the day after they arrived, my mother said, "Daddy's sort of out of it. He's still exhausted from the trip."

Well, my father stayed sort of out of it. In fact, he got more and more out of it. Day by day he slipped further and further away from us into a world of silence leaving us alienated, frustrated and anguished. When his ability to talk left him, he used facial gestures and hand motions to communicate. His deteriorating mind remained trapped within a body that still functioned.

Our family tried to pull my father back. We believed that this could be done by sheer force of will on our part. We tried to think up ways to anchor my father to this world. We'd go on a trip; build a deck together; read to him from the newspapers and from books; and we'd show him family photos—anything to keep his mind alert. But all of these efforts proved futile; nothing we did would ever bring him back to the way he was.

Through all the downhill months, my mother cared for him. She fed him when he couldn't feed himself any longer, she showered him, she shaved him. When he became incontinent, she cleaned him and changed him and washed up after him. It was mentally and physically exhausting and it soon got to a point at which she was in severe need of relief. The toll that the caregiving was taking on her caused us to actually fear for her health; taking care of him was making her ill. She needed time off and someone to help her—someone who was able to keep my father's mind active and working to the best of its ability.

My mother often said that she could have kept my father home with her until the end of his life if only she had been able to have help during the day—some time for herself and some sort of stimulating activity for her husband. Near the end of my father's life, we brought him for an evaluation to Burke Institute in White Plains, New York. We were astounded to discover that Burke, in fact, had a place that might have helped both my father in the form of an adult day care center. Unfortunately, by the time we learned about it, my father had regressed beyond the point where a day-care setting would have helped him.

Daily, weekly and monthly, I get phone calls from beleaguered and caring families who are looking for the relief that an adult day-care center can offer. I hear stories that parallel in many ways the one I've just told. Often I'll hear, "she just sits staring at the walls" or, "there has to be something else for him to do but watch 18 hours of television a day" or, "the only time she seems to be like her old self is when we have company over."

Families tell stories about once vibrant parents, siblings and aunts who can't remember recent events and whom the family fears to leave home alone during the day. They tell of the promises they made "never to put him in a home." They tell familiar tales of their loved ones increasing confusion and how they—the family—are more and more at a loss as to how to cope. I am continually astounded with the lack of information—virtually no knowledge that the possibility of an adult day care center exists. In fact, families more often stumble upon us than seek us out.

The history of adult day care in the United States is a recent one. Its model is the English day hospital and it was adopted here in the 1970s through very limited government funding. In 1970 there were perhaps 15 adult day care centers in the entire U.S. Now there are thousands, although this continues to be a fairly well-kept secret.

There are three general kinds of adult day care:

- social (provides only social interaction, for the purpose of resocialization)

- preventive maintenance/medical (provides health care maintenance, for the purpose of medical intervention, if appropriate)
- day treatment (provides more intensive medical or psychiatric treatment)

Some adult day centers are one kind or a combination of kinds, and some have started as one and become another, mostly as a result of changes in clientele. Adult day care has always needed to chase funding streams. Therefore, if an Alzheimer's grant suddenly became available, the day center courted Alzheimer's victims.

In 1975, funding from Title XX (part of the Older Americans Act) was the only money available to support adult day care. Since the Title XX money dried up quite early in day care history, many adult day care programs began to seek other funding mechanisms. (As an example of how meager Title XX funds continue to be, we currently receive $18 per client per day from Title XX. Our private pay members, on the other hand, are paying a more realistic $45 per day.) The adult day care program at Daughters of Israel Geriatric Center is funded by seven different sources. Each county and state has its own criteria and its own programs, but in Essex County, New Jersey, our members are paid for by (1) Title XX, (2) a New Jersey Department of Health gerontology grant, (3) an Essex County respite grant and (4) four separate Medicaid programs. The clear advantage of having multiple sources of funding is that formerly ineligible clients now have several options for reimbursement. Unfortunately, accessing these various sources of funding involves a major time commitment to ensure compliance with varying documentation requirements.

Our center and others like ours provide a warm, enveloping environment for the frail elderly. We have on our staff nurses, recreational therapists, a social worker, a supervising dietitian and a medical director. We provide transportation in small buses and vans. All of our drivers cater to the special needs of our elderly population. Our drivers are part of the day center team. They serve in the front line as our reconnaissance. Often they are the ones to provide us with the earliest information on changes in a client may be exhibiting.

The day center is peopled with members in all stages of mental acuity. For the most able, we provide trips and entertainment which keeps them informed and independent. For those clients who are most confused, we provide equally interesting programming, but the activities are geared to their level of ability.

As an example, we took a ride on the Staten Island Ferry to observe the bustle of New York harbor. This was an activity for our more capable day center participants. Negotiating stairs, knowing where to sit and when to walk around, understanding where the bathrooms are, remembering where our staff members are sitting, knowing to stay seated when the boat is docking—these are abilities that not all of our clients still possess.

For the less able we have shorter trips that enable them to get out without putting them at risk. We stress the abilities they still have. A trip down memory lane to various neighborhoods in Newark (where most of our people grew up), an afternoon in the park picnicking and feeding ducks, a trip to see the cherry blossoms in bloom—these trips can all be negotiated and enjoyed by our more confused members.

In years past, the choice of how to best help a disoriented or demented loved one was limited. With resources—a large home, a large income, a large family—the fortunate few were often able to keep someone at home until the end of their lives. However, the rosy picture of a family cheerily chipping in to help a grandfather in his final days is largely the stuff of fantasy. The truth is that for everyone it was always an unbearably hard situation fraught with resentment and frustration.

In the 1990s we are more fortunate because there now exists a continuum of care for the elderly. Families have options that didn't exist before. Because of the services offered by support service apartment houses, congregate living programs and adult day care centers, no longer is there only one choice—the a nursing home. We are allowing people to remain in the community for as long as possible by providing viable alternatives to institutionalization.

For those who are caring for an increasingly confused family member, we offer a way to continue to provide that care. Families know that their relatives are being safely cared for. They can go on with their own lives—working, socializing, shopping—and be able to face life with renewed resolve because of the services we provide.

A day in our center begins with a buffet breakfast. Because many of our members come only a few times a week, our multidisciplinary team uses the morning meal as a time to evaluate changes in members. Morning activities begin with a synopsis of the day's news and exercises geared to the age and ability of our population. The current day's activities are discussed. We also have two large bulletin boards listing the events that will take place during that day. One lists all the events, the other highlights that day's special event. These serve to remind our clients who are unable to retain new information about what is going on during the day.

We take our members food shopping twice a week and to a mall, thrift shops and discount stores once a month. We provide to those clients who go shopping the freedom of choice in a life where their options are increasingly diminished.

In our constant attempt to promote and maintain independence, the day center runs a sheltered workshop several times a week. Those members who wish to participate do simple packaging and are paid per piece. This activity provides socialization for the worker/clients and a sense of continued worth, since the packaging job is uncomplicated enough for almost all of our members to succeed. Further, because of the remuneration they receive, our clients have a sense of retaining skills that are still of monetary value.

Since even the most disoriented clients are able to get value out of singing, we schedule a singalong at least once a week. We find that if we stick to songs that are old and therefore familiar, every one of our members can join in. For those of our people who are less impaired, we have an active choral group that goes out at least once a month to entertain at other nursing homes, day centers and women's groups. They are always met with enthusiasm and are often videotaped by their hosts. This feeds the healthy ego needs of people often sorely missing concrete reminders of their present worth to society.

Our day center at Daughters of Israel Geriatric Center began 16 years ago and was at that time catering to a younger and more capable clientele. The client of yesterday now more appropriately attends a senior citizen drop-in center. The new members we get are coming to us older and more mentally and physically debilitated. In fact, 16 years ago the people we now attend to on an outpatient basis, would have then been considered as nursing home-appropriate. Some of our members, even the first day they arrive, seem only a step away from nursing home placement. Our goal is to try to make that step as long a one as possible. The more we can delay or prevent premature institutionalization, the more we see ourselves succeeding.

Our staff is in constant contact with families, physicians and social agencies to inform them of what we observe at the day center. We have weekly staff meetings to discuss our clients in order to track each member's status.

Because over 60 percent of our population has some form of diagnosed dementia, we build into our schedule special discussion groups, each geared to the level of confusion of its participants. For clients beyond reality orientation, we lead validation therapy sessions. We also conduct life review activities groups, which are very successful because although short-term memory is often lost, the long-term memory of most of our clients has been left unimpaired.

The elderly who attend the adult day center at Daughters of Israel are particularly fortunate because ours is a progressive-thinking agency with an attitude that encourages its staff to try new things. The minds of the employees are always being stretched and our clients surely benefit from this.

As an example, when we found ourselves with more leftovers from lunch and breakfast than we could store, we broached the subject with our administrator of selling whole meals for 25 cents each. The money realized from the sale of this food now goes through Save the Children Federation to support needy children. We specifically indicated our desire to help American inner-city children. It pleases our members enormously to know that they, many of whom grew up in poor city neighborhoods themselves, are now able to help children in need. At the members' suggestion, we are sending donations to other mainstream charities as well.

When our day center began 16 years ago, virtually all day center participants were obliged to pay their own way. Now the complete opposite is true. The income-based entitlements of the state and county agencies mentioned earlier fund the attendance of virtually all of our members. In addition, we belong to a program called the New Jersey Food Bank which allows us to purchase, for pennies a pound, unsold, overstocked and discontinued foods. Once a week we are able to send home with our members home a large shopping bag full of groceries at no charge to them. This, in addition to the large breakfast and lunch we serve, enables us to feel safe that our clients whose families supervise them from afar are well fed.

With dignity and care, our day center is daily reinforcing the self-worth of its participants. We are helping families in the yeoman task they've set for themselves: to keep their family members at home as long as possible. It is the proud task of those who work in adult day care centers to help achieve that goal.

6

Meeting the Dental Needs
of the Elderly

Mayra Suero-Wade, DDS, MPH

The elderly population is presently gaining attention within the dental profession. For years, many dentists have been reluctant to treat the elderly population because it was believed that the elderly were not concerned about their dental health, or that their medical complications were unmanageable, or that they were unable to afford dental care (Evans 1984). These beliefs are changing and today many dentists are reaching out to the elderly. According to Dr. Linda Niessen, a public health specialist in geriatric dentistry, the focus is now on treatment modes for the older patient. One of the reasons for this is that the characteristics of the U.S. population are changing; people are getting older and there is a trend to continue looking and feeling the best possible. The elderly today are keeping their teeth longer and are seeking dental care in increasing numbers. Studies of vital statistics in 1979 have shown that less than half (45 percent) of the elderly population is edentulous (Kelly 1989). This number is probably lower today.

Demographic studies (ADA 1982) show that 29 million persons were aged 65 and older in 1986, accounting for approximately 12 percent of the total population. Population experts predict that the current trend is likely to continue in the future; by the year 2000 it is projected that there will be approximately 34 million individuals aged 65 and over, or roughly 13 percent of the population. Moderate growth of this age group is expected to continue until the end of the first decade of the 21st century when the number of older adults will soar as the baby boom generation reaches retirement age (ADA 1982; Geboy 1985). The estimated U.S. Government figures predict that 75 percent of dental patients will be over 65 years of age within 20 years (Special Committee on Aging 1983).

To ensure oral health and quality dental care for the elderly, proper planning to meet the dental treatment needs of this group is important. With longer retention of teeth there is increased prevalence of dental-related problems. The data are not conclusive, but they suggest that root caries, periodontal disease and prosthetic needs will increase as well (Beck 1983).

In order to properly serve this group, a method for examination, diagnosis, treatment, prevention and maintenance should be tailor-made for the elderly patient. In addition, there are economic, psychological and physical barriers that must be addressed in order to increase the access and availability of dental services to the elderly (Antczak and Branch 1985).

SENIOR DENTAL CARE STUDY

Materials and Methods

A group of 22 senior citizens, all over 55 years of age, were surveyed. All of them were members of the Lutheran Church meal program in New York City. A questionnaire was distributed to all seniors at the program's center after permission was granted from management and an explanation of the study was given. Participation was on a volunteer basis. The questionnaire composed of five yes/no and seven open-ended questions, was filled out independently by most of the participants. Four respondents required help and their responses were collected in an interview. The participants were of similar socioeconomic background, lived in the same neighborhood and were divided equally into males and females.

Results

Of the 22 respondents questioned, only 32 percent (7) saw a dentist on a regular basis (less than once per year for a check-up or prophylactic care), 22 percent (5) had been to the dentist within 6 months, and 72 percent (16) felt they had specific dental needs (e.g. restorations, prosthetic or periodontic needs) that were neglected. Fifty-five percent of respondents felt there was a need for dental care. Sixty-eight percent of the respondents felt that lack of dental care limited some physical or social function. There were indications that financial constraint and lack of dental insurance restricted dental care for some of the elderly. This was evident when

36 percent of the respondents said they could not afford dental care and 91 percent said that if Medicare covered part of their dental expenses, they would visit the dentist when they needed care. Though most of the elderly questioned attested to living on restricted incomes, 86 percent (19 out of 22) of respondents had to pay for dental care out of pocket.

Discussion

The data collected was in accordance with a Massachusetts study (Antczak and Branch 1964) that investigated dental care barriers experienced by the elderly. It was found in this study that 30 percent of the respondents utilized dental services and 70 percent of the respondents required dental treatment but were not receiving it due to lack of dental coverage and other physical and psychological restraints. In another study Berkey and colleagues (1985) showed that there is a high correlation between dental problems and negative physical and social effects. The data from the New York study confirmed Berkey's findings, which showed that speech and eating impairment was common among elderly with dental problems.

TOWARD BETTER GERIATRIC DENTAL CARE

Studies continue to identify the problems encountered by the elderly in need of dental care. A sensible plan of evaluation and treatment should be put together to start an effective solution process. First of all, the concept of treating the elderly should be holistic; in other words, the patient and his individual external influences must be taken into account. One of the most important aspects of providing proper care to the elderly is obtaining a complete history (medical, drug, dental and psychosocial). A team approach is necessary (consultation with other health professionals in contact with the patient and if appropriate also with the family). This will allow proper assessment of the drug, mental, physical and disease status of the patient.

The *medical and drug histories* should be thorough, taking into account that the elderly population overall have higher incidence and prevalence rates of chronic diseases. This will sometimes mean that the elderly patient is taking multiple medications (Picozzi and Neidle 1984), some of which may be contributing to oral disease. An example is the xerostomia (dry-mouth) caused by diazepam, antihistamines, anticholinergic drugs and diuretic therapy with water restriction (Shafer et al. 1983). If one knows the patient is taking any of these medications, some of the effects of xerostomia (root caries, periodontal disease) can be prevented or decreased with use of a salivary substitute and proper oral hygiene. If antibiotic prophylaxis is needed, one should check that the appropriate antibiotic regimen is given to the patient (Committee on Rheumatic Fever 1985).

Drug interactions such as competition, synergism or antagonism are important to know; it will help prevent overmedication, cumulation or toxic reactions to drugs (Lamy 1986). The elderly have a heightened sensitivity to certain drugs. One must remember that a geriatric patient may need lower doses of a drug than a younger patient. A therapeutic level can be achieved with lower doses because of altered drug distribution, altered metabolism and decreased renal excretion (Lamy 1986). As a result, lower doses of local anesthetics may be used. One should be cautious of using epinephrine in local anesthesia because of its systemic effects on hypertension and its thyrotoxic effect on hyperthyroidism (Wells et al. 1980). Instead of using narcotic agents such as codeine for post-surgical pain relief, aspirin may be used effectively, but it too has contraindications (GI disorders) and its competition with other drugs (coumarin anticoagulant, oral hypoglycemic agents) for the same plasma protein binding site may cause bleeding problems.

Dental and psychosocial histories also provide pertinent information for treatment planning. One must know about a patient's dental awareness and also about the nature of his compliance to treatment and home care. Questions about oral hygiene, nutrition, past dental experiences and how the patient feels about dental treatment will give the dentist information about the patient's likes and dislikes (see chart at end of chapter). It is also important to determine a patients extent of dental education as well as if he is apprehensive or anxious, compliant or resistant. Open communication with patients about their needs and their wants will be helpful in providing individualized dental treatment.

Examination of the patient should include the entire head and neck area. The presence of a recent set of radiographs and models will aid in diagnosis and planning. During examination it is important to recognize the difference between age-related oral changes and disease-related changes. Atrophy of mucous membranes and gingival recession may be normal findings in a patient who is over 65 years old because of decrease in connective tissue and cell function (Levy and Konigsberg 1974). On the other hand, if tissue atrophy is accompanied by itching, redness or burning, or if recession is present along with mobility of the teeth and significant pocket depth, this indicates a disease state. All the nodes in the head and neck should also be inspected. Abnormal nodes (enlarged firm or tender) may be signs of infection or cancer. The thyroid gland should be checked for normal size and the temporomandibular joint (TMJ) area should be checked for any abnormal symptoms.

Dentistry cannot be based on standardized treatment and if it is it will only lead to disappointments and failures. Patients of the same physiologic age, say 70 years, may have different needs based on their health status. A healthy, independent 70 year old will have different treatment needs than a frail person of the same age. Effective planning and treating must also consider a patients handicaps or limitations. Only after review of the patient's overall state of health should the treatment plan be considered.

Preventive dental treatment should be part of the geriatric patient's care. It has been shown that older patients accumulate plaque at a faster rate and in greater quantities than younger patients (Holm-Pedersen 1975). Plaque is a common etiologic factor of caries and periodontal disease. Proper plaque control is a must for the elderly patient. For this reason dental education should be given concurrent with dental treatment to increase oral health and decrease failure of treatment. Instruction and encouragement on how to use home care dental aids is very important. Oral hygiene instructions should include the following: interproximal flossing, proper brushing (teeth, gingiva, and tongue) with a soft tooth brush, and inspection of teeth after cleaning. Clean teeth will have open embrasures (air flows easily between teeth). Clean teeth will make a squeaky sound when floss is used interproximally. Running a clean finger on the facial or lingual surfaces of clean teeth will also produce a squeaky sound. Fluoride treatments should be recommended to patients with high caries rates, or decreased salivary flow and patients undergoing head and neck cancer therapy.

After the completion of treatment, the patient should be placed on a maintenance/assessment program to monitor oral health and observe for any new developing problem. Recall can be set between 3 and 6 months depending on the patient's risk for caries or periodontal status (mobility, inflammation, sensitivity, etc.). A recall session should include an examination, an update of radiographs, if needed and a "prophy" and a fluoride treatment. If the patient needs further treatment, it should be arranged immediately.

INCREASING DENTAL CARE UTILIZATION

The dental profession is doing what it can to address the needs of the elderly, but the elderly's dental care utilization rate is still the lowest of any group, with the exception of children below the age of 6 (Antczak and Branch 1985). The dental profession must focus their attention on removing the existing barriers that limit the availability and accessibility of dental care to the elderly. These barriers can be considered in three categories: physical, psychological and financial.

Physical barriers can be overcome with the implementation of structural changes to the dental facility: ramps and wide doorways for those in wheelchairs, hand rails in rest rooms and in long hallways and adaptable dental chairs for the physically impaired. The dentist must also be equipped with an updated emergency kit and know current cardiopulmonary resuscitation (CPR) techniques.

Psychological barriers come from the patient as well as from the dentist. Patients may be fearful of dental treatment due to past experiences or they may not be aware of their need for dental care. Of the respondents I questioned, 45 percent felt they did not need dental care, but when asked about whether they had specific dental problems, 72 percent responded positively, demonstrating the disparity between want and need. On the other hand, the dentist may also have preconceived ideas of elderly patients and treat them as a group rather than as individuals. After working with the elderly I discovered that each individual must be approached with care and sensitivity. They are concerned about details and want to know every aspect of their treatment. The feelings and concerns of the elderly are similar to those of young adults: they want to look good and feel good. Psychological barriers and misconceptions limit the patient-provider relationship. Getting rid of these barriers through education will enhance communication on both sides.

Last is the topic of *economic barriers*. This is a complicated subject when it comes to the elderly because while seniors as a whole are the wealthiest segment of our population, a significant portion of elderly people are on a fixed income and do not have dental coverage under the Medicare plan. The addition of dental services to the Medicare program will decrease financial barriers for the elderly. However, it is unlikely that dental coverage will be provided when the national budgetary focus is presently on reducing health expenditures. Recently there has been a push from the medical and dental professions to put pressure on government to increase Medicare benefits, but no solutions have been found as yet. The dental community might have to take charge of this situation and find alternative ways to eliminate the economic barriers that exist for those who cannot afford dental care.

Model programs such as Kaiser and the Ultracare Program in California (Marcus et al. 1984) have been successful in including comprehensive dental care in their health benefit package. These pilot programs are sponsored by the federal Health Care Financing Administration. In health maintenance organizations (HMOs), patients pay a yearly fee for all their health needs. Fees are based on projections of utilization of services. However, HMOs were designed for the provision of only medical, not dental, care and education (Donaldson et al. 1985).

Development of a dental maintenance organization can complement and supply the dental care needs that are left out by some HMOs. Another innovative method of increasing dental care utilization for populations on fixed incomes is by installing an "in-office" dental insurance program. With this program the patient pays the doctor a yearly set fee to receive all preventive and certain restorative services.

DENTAL SERVICES FOR THE HOMEBOUND AND INSTITUTIONALIZED

A historically acknowledged access barrier to dental care for certain population groups is the inability to get to the dentist's office. Among these are individuals who are institutionalized or homebound. This lack of mobility translates into a lack of health care that has serious human consequences. Patients in long-term care and individuals who are homebound often must experience pain and the spread of oral infection before care is provided.

To make dental care accessible to the homebound or institutionalized elderly, technologically updated portable dental units are available (Berkey and Douglass 1987). It is now possible to transport and operate these portable units in a very efficient manner. Dentists who are involved in providing this type of dental service have found both psychological and financial rewards (Teer 1989).

"Dentistry in Motion," a mobile dentistry service, is a new and innovative approach to meet the needs of both the homebound and the institutionalized individual. These functionally dependent persons have special needs that have been identified by Ettinger and Miller-Eldridge (1985). They found that only 18 percent of nursing homes provided any type of regular dental care, that the average number of years elapsing since a resident's last dental visit was 8 years, that 80 percent of patients in long-term care facilities need extensive dental treatment and that approximately 50 percent of nursing home patients are confined to their rooms. An option such as "Dentistry in Motion" strives to meet the needs of those who cannot get to the dental office by bringing the office to the institution or the home.

This service also addresses the availability of dental care to other types of individuals who cannot access the dental office, such as persons residing in a retirement community, the homeless and the medically disfranchised. This last group has been thought to include persons who are medically knowledgeable, but do not seek and may not even want medical or dental care. This is a misconception; the main reason for their behavior is that medical and dental care has not been made available to them in the past. Mobile dentistry is designed to increase the availability of dental care to those who are not receiving it. This group is in tremendous need of dental care supervision; candidiasis, hairy leukoplakia and periodontal disease are conditions found in high frequency. In addition, since this population is at risk for HIV infection and because the mouth often shows the first clinical signs of HIV, an oral examination may provide early detection and management. Another misconception about this group is that dental care is not a priority for them. On the contrary, oral health is a part of every person's sense of being healthy. The ability to participate in and enjoy social activities and meals is greatly dependent upon oral health. Therefore, it is important to teach basic hygiene of the oral environment to maintain general good health.

Several misconceptions exist about mobile dentistry, including the concept that services are performed in a van, that the equipment is bulky and that the equipment used is less powerful than that found in dental offices. "Dentistry in Motion" brings its equipment into the facility or home and into a room that is convenient for the patient. It can even be placed beside a bed for those who are bedridden. The latest in compactness and design, it can be transported in a car and set-up takes only 5 minutes. This state-of-the-art equipment is engineered to have the power to serve all the dental care needs of the patient. The array of services provided includes gross examination, cleaning, x-rays, diagnosis, restoration of carious lesions, provision and repair of dentures, follow-up and emergency care, emergency care and comprehensive new admission examinations for those entering a long-term care facility.

DETERMINING THE NEED OF DENTAL CARE
IN THE SENIOR CITIZEN POPULATION

Your Name: _____

1. Do you see a dentist on a regular basis? _____
2. Do you see a medical doctor regularly? _____
3. When was the last time you visited a dentist for care?

       specific date _____
  _____ less than 6 months ago
  _____ 1 year ago
  _____ 2 years ago
  _____ more than 2 years ago

4. Do you feel you need dental care? _____

5. What type of dental care do you feel you need?
        (check all that apply)

_____ Need a professional cleaning of teeth and gums (periodontist)
_____ Need fillings - restorations of carious teeth
_____ Need replacement of missing teeth (denture or fix bridge)
_____ Need to improve home care (oral hygiene instructions)
_____ Need repair of present dentures
_____ Need cleaning of dentures
_____ Other dental care, please specify: _____

6. If you have not been to the dentist for dental care (within the last year), what was the reason for not going? (check all that apply)

_____ No transportation
_____ Couldn't afford dental care
_____ Didn't know a dentist in the area
_____ Didn't need dental care
_____ Other reason, please specify: _____

7. Does the lack of dental care affect any of the following functions?

_____ Eating
_____ Speaking
_____ Socializing
_____ Affects other functions, please specify: _____

8. How do you (or would you) pay for dental care when visiting a dentist?

_____ Pay with own savings
_____ Pay with insurance
_____ Pay from savings and insurance
_____ Medicaid
_____ Other, specify: _____

9. Has lack of finance ever stopped you from getting dental care?_____

10. If Medicare covered part of your dental expenses would you go to the dentist?

11. Do you clean your teeth on a regular basis? _____

12. How often do you clean your teeth?

REFERENCES

American Dental Association: Interim Report of the American Dental Association's Special Committee on the Future of Dentistry, Chicago, 1982.

Antczak, A.A. and L.G. Branch. Perceived barriers to the use of dental services by the elderly. *Gerodontics* 4:194-198, 1985.

Beck, J.D. The epidemiology of dental disease in the elderly. *Gerotondology* 3(1):5-13, 1984.

Berkey, D.B., R.L. Call and M.L. Lope. Oral health perceptions and self-esteem in non-institutionalized older adults. *Gerodontics* 4:213-216, 1985.

Berkey, B. and R. Douglass. Improving dental access for the nursing home resident: portable dentistry intervention. *Gerodontics* 3(6):266-268, 1987.

Committee on rheumatic fever and infective endocarditis. *J. Am. Dent. Assoc.* 110:98-100, 1985.

Donaldson, M.S., J.A. Nichlason and J.E. Ott. Needs-based health promotion program serves as HMO marketing tool. *Public Health Rep.* 100(3):270-277, May-June 1985.

Evans, R.W. The aging dental patient: myths and reality. *Gerodontology* 3(4):271-273, 1984.

Geboy, M.J. *Communication and Behavior Management in Dentistry.* Baltimore: Williams & Wilkins, 1985.

Holm-Pedersen, P., N. Agerbek and E. Theilade. Experimental gingivitis in young and elderly individuals. *J. Clin. Periodontics* 2:14-24, 1975.

Kelly, J.E. Basic Data on Dental Examination Findings of Persons 1-74 Years. United States Vital Statistics and Health Survey No. 214. DHEW Publication No. 79-11662, 1979.

Lamy, P.P. The elderly and drug interactions. *J. Am. Geriatric Soc.* 34(8): 586-592, 1986.

Levy, B.M. and I. Konigsberg. Gerontology and the practice of geriatric dentistry. *Gerodontology* 3(4):255-257, 1974.

Marcus, M., M.H. Schoen and S. May. An alternative method for financing care for the non-institutionalized geriatric dental Patient. *Gerodontology* 3(4):219-224, 1984.

Picozzi, A. and E.A. Neidle. Geriatric pharmacology for the dentist. *Dent. Clin. North Am.* 28(3):581-591, 1984.

Report of the Special Committee on Aging, United States Senate. *Developments in Aging, 1982.* Washington DC: U.S. Government Printing Office, 1983.

Shafer, W.G., M.K. Hine and B.M. Levy. *A Textbook of Oral Pathology, 4th Ed.* Philadelphia: W.B. Saunders, 1983.

Sonkin, S. Financing dental care for older Americans in the 21st century. *Gerodontics* 4:291-293, 1985.

Teer, L. Special delivery...mobile dentist is moved by patients. *UMDNJ Health State* 7(1):36, Spring 1989.

Wells, J.E., M.W. Reed and V.M. Coury. *Review of Basic Science and Clinical Dentistry,* Vol. 2, Philadelphia: Lippincott, 1980.

7

Respite Care for the Visually Impaired and Their Families

Nancy D. Weber, MSSW, ACSW
and Pamela Schneider, MSW, CSW

Mrs. D, an 85-year-old blind woman who lives with her caregiver daughter, enjoyed a 12-day overnight residential recreation program at Vacation Camp for the Blind while receiving personal care assistance. Shortly after her mother's return, the daughter arranged for a temporary private home care worker to stay with her mother while she attended a business trip. The day before she was due to leave, the home care worker suddenly canceled. The daughter called the camp and arranged for her mother to return for another session while she was out of town.

A legally blind woman in her seventies, Mrs. L had been attending Vacation Camp for the Blind for many years. One summer she did not return and the staff called to find out why. She explained that her sighted husband was now too ill to be left home alone. With the help and encouragement of the staff, she decided to speak to her daughter about caring for the father temporarily so that she could take a needed break. Mrs. L convinced her daughter and used the camp for her own rest and renewal, returning home to care for her sick husband for the remainder of the year.

These two examples illustrate the need that exists and a solution that has been successfully employed by a program, Vacation Camp for the Blind, serving elderly blind and multiply handicapped persons and their families.

NEED FOR RESPITE CARE SERVICES

Respite care services are one response to the long-term care and home care crisis in the United States today as individual needs outpace the resources to meet them. The rapidly growing elderly frail and disabled population is creating pressure on policymakers, legislators, health care services, insurers, corporations and families, and on elderly and disabled persons themselves. In a 1984-85 census study, 13.5 million people in the United States identified themselves as having a severe disability (*New York Times*, December 1986). The rate of disability increases with age with more than half of persons 65 years and older who report a disability that effects their daily functioning. An estimated 65 million people or nearly 22 percent of the American population will be 65 years or older by the year 2030.

According to the 1987 National Medical Expenditure Survey an estimated 9.5 million noninstitutionalized persons (4 percent of the population) experience difficulty in performing everyday basic life activities due to mental or physical health problems. A total of 5.6 million persons reporting difficulty are age 65 and older, a 20.1 percentage of the total population in that age group. At ages 85 and older, 1.3 million individuals (57.6 percent of the total population of 2.2 million persons 85 or older) experience difficulty performing basic life activities (Disability Statistics Abstract, 1992).

One of the most common disabling conditions experienced by older persons is vision impairment. It has been noted that "age is the most powerful predictor of the prevalence of blindness and visual impairment" (Lowman and Kirchner 1979). Approximately 10 to 15 percent of the overall elderly population is severely visually impaired. Elderly persons with severe vision impairment (defined as inability to read regular print even with glasses or acuity of 20/70 in the better eye with correction) constitute nearly 80 percent of the total population of persons with severe visual impairment. (Orr 1992; Weber 1991). It is estimated that severely visually impaired older people in the United States will increase from over 2 million in 1980, to 3.2 million in the year 2000, to an estimated 4.6. million in the year 2020. The population age 85 and over, where prevalence of severe visual impairment is one in four, will number 1.6 million in the year 2010, meaning an estimated 400,000 severely visually impaired persons over the age of 85 (Crews 1991).

Most elderly people and most people who are visually impaired do not require the daily assistance of someone in their home. But like Mrs. D, approximately 12 percent of all older people living in the community require daily home care assistance. Three out of four elderly people, like Mrs. L and her husband, depend exclusively on spouses, children, other relatives and friends for this care (Soldo 1985).

The absolute numbers of older people are increasing rapidly. An increase in the elderly population does not necessarily imply that most will be sick or dependent (Brody 1981). However, mental and physical impairments that lead to dependency do increase with age. There is now a greater likelihood of two generations of elderly persons in one family in need of some care. There has been an increase in the old caring for the very old, highlighting the vulnerability of all generations when a caregiver becomes incapacitated (Troll et al. 1979; Fengler and Goodrich 1979; Brubaker 1983).

FAMILY CAREGIVING

> Mr. M, a 43-year-old blind, developmentally disabled, multiply handicapped man with limited verbal skills, lives with his 78-year-old mother. His mother had also been caring for his terminally ill father who died just before the summer camp season. His mother asked if her son could stay at Vacation Camp for the Blind for 3 sessions (6 weeks) instead of just 1. In addition, two camp staff volunteered to extend the respite care by staying with him at camp during the 2 weekend breaks between sessions. His mother needed the time to recover from her loss and did not know how to explain to her son that his father had died. The camp staff along with his mother, who came to camp for visits, encouraged him to talk about "Daddy" and told him that Daddy would not be visiting anymore and that he had died and was in heaven. The staff listened to his constant statements and questions, reinforcing the new information. He received one-to-one attention and over time his questioning decreased. Although not sure if he completely understood the information about his father's death, by the end of the summer his mother felt able to have him return home.

It is emotionally stressful and burdensome for many families to provide care at home for an older or disabled person. In the example of Mr. M, stress was created for his elderly mother not only because of the responsibility for his care, but also because of the additional care she provided for her terminally ill spouse and the eventual need to tell her son about his father's death.

Stress has been defined as the nonspecific response of the body to any demand made upon it that feels as if it cannot be handled (Selye 1974). Stress can be perceived as an imbalance between a demand and the ability to respond, a sense of overload. The intensity and the duration will fluctuate. A particular condition or similar situation may be perceived as stressful by some persons and not by others. Even when people describe a similar perception of stress, they often react differently. Family adaptive techniques and history are factors in the perception of stress. Individuals and families manifest and respond to stress in different ways (McCubbin et al. 1983) and effectively cope with stress to varying degrees.

Caregiving leads to many different reactions. Some of the most negative types of stress reported by caregivers include stress related to carrying out multiple roles such as caregiver, spouse or parent; exhaustion; tension; neglect of other family members; resentment; frustration; lack of time for chores or leisure pursuits; financial burdens; inconvenience; reported increase in anxiety; depression; and rivalry between family members (Silverstone and Hyman 1978; Crossman et al. 1981; Frankfather et al. 1981; Miller 1981; Brody 1981; Horowitz and Dobrof 1982; Kayser 1984; Isett 1984; Cohen and Warren 1985; Pennsylvania Department of Aging 1986).

Families continue to provide care, despite experiences and research to demonstrate how difficult it is. There are many reasons given by family caregivers as to why they continue to endure the stress of providing care. These include guilt, obligation, satisfaction, gratification, appreciation, affection, positive family and intergenerational relations, expectations, reciprocity, desire to avoid institutional or nursing home placement at all costs and filial responsibility (Brody 1981; Horowitz and Dobrof 1982; Perlman 1983; Cicerelli 1983; Kayser 1984; Cohen and Warren 1985; Kingson et al. 1986). Positive and negative feelings often coexist in the same relationship, and even when conflict exists, it does not necessarily interfere with helping behavior (Brubaker 1983).

Most caregivers are women, usually spouses, daughters or siblings (Horowitz 1985; Horowitz and Dobrof 1982; Snyder and Keefe 1985). However, changes in the modern family are creating circumstances that seriously affect the family caregiver of the future, and the extent to which this role will be possible. More women are working outside the home; therefore they may be less available or under even greater stress when they do provide care. Many women are returning to the work force or advancing in their careers just when they are more likely to be needed to care for a dependent parent or spouse. Divorce is more common. Families are becoming smaller and there will be fewer children able to provide for their "baby boom" parents. Older people with no children have been at greater risk for institutional and nursing home placements. As couples of the 1990s chose not to have any children, to have fewer children and to delay having children, they are rarely thinking ahead, acknowledging and accepting the greater risk of living in a nursing home in their old age.

THE FAMILY AS A SYSTEM

A "deinstitutionalized," blind, multiply handicapped woman, Miss R, lived with her mother who was in her late seventies. The daughter had been abused in the past and would not allow her mother to leave her with anyone else. Her mother found out that she had been diagnosed with cancer and she desperately needed a rest and time to accept the news of her own medical problems. Miss R and her mother attended Vacation Camp for the Blind together for one 12-day session. During the day, at first Miss R participated in activities only when her mother was present and then more frequently without her. For the following 2 summers, the mother attended with her daughter initially but was able to leave for longer periods and eventually was able to leave her daughter completely in the care of the camp staff for a few days and then for a full week. At first, Miss R had repeated tantrums, would not feed herself and had frequent toileting accidents. These behaviors were common at home whenever there was a change in routine. She received one-to-one care for 24 hours a day from the camp staff. After 2 summers her mother was finally able to get a full break of 12 days, knowing that her daughter was receiving quality care. The mother's cancer is currently in remission.

A couple in their eighties came to camp with their daughter, Miss S, a 41-year-old, blind woman with Down syndrome. Both parents have serious heart conditions and arthritis. They were reluctant to have anyone else take care of their daughter but they were exhausted and knew that they needed a rest. They attended Vacation Camp for the Blind together as a family and at first took turns staying with their daughter at activities. After 5 days they allowed the staff to bring her to activities without them. While at camp, the staff helped them to locate a daytime respite program in their neighborhood at home and began the process of considering long range plans for Miss S when they were no longer able to care for her.

As we learn about family caregiving and study primary caregivers, it is important to address the whole family as a system (Troll et al. 1979; Brubaker 1983). The caregiving parents of both Miss R and Miss S need the break from daily caregiving but need time to withdraw from the daily care to help themselves and their children adjust to the change gradually. Family members influence one another. Families have the unique ability to mediate the reactions and encourage coping behaviors of other family members in times of change, crisis and stress (Kaplan et al. 1973). When individuals are part of families, they often do not resolve their own problems independently. Yet if the crisis or stress is great enough and sufficiently prolonged, the role of the family as a buffer can falter. The physical and emotional needs and demands that a dependent person makes on the primary caregiver and other family members create a family crisis that includes the caregiver and the care receiver. As demands on the family increase, such as when the dependent person's needs increase, the family system readjusts. Caregiver stress is family stress. Caregiver coping is family coping. Dynamics around caregiving are influenced by a family's previous history of crisis management. The stress model of family functioning in the face of a crisis depicts the family as a system of complementary roles. Either the family will absorb the stress or succumb to it. The capacity for sustaining care regardless of the age or type of disability of the dependent person is also influenced by cultural and social factors (Perlman 1983). Dependent persons, their caregivers and families do not always agree on the type of care needed and can differ in their experience of being a part of a caregiving family (Frankfather et al. 1981).

By viewing the family as a system, with reactions to one another's emotional states, a blueprint is offered for understanding the dependent person and the caregiver. Pressures or constraints on any one family member will impinge on all other role relationships within the family (Troll et al. 1979; McCubbin et al. 1983). Stress experienced by any member of the family will affect all other family members.

RESPITE CARE: HISTORY, FUNDING AND STRUCTURE

Respite care is physical, emotional or social care of a dependent person by someone other than the primary caregiver in order to provide the latter with a temporary reprieve or relief from caregiving tasks and duties. First specifically named and developed in Europe in the 1960s, respite care has been identified by gerontologists and researchers on caregiving and stress as one approach to giving needed support to family caregivers (Horowitz and Dobrof 1982; Kayser 1984; Snyder and Keefe 1985; Cohen and Warren 1985). Respite care services vary according to locale, agency resources and family needs. Respite or relief care can be offered for an hour, several hours, a day, several days, weekends, or several weeks at a time. Respite may be offered at specific intervals each week on a long-term basis. The earliest respite care services were available to families of mentally retarded or developmentally disabled persons. Development of respite for the families of this population was supported in New York State by the normalization and deinstitutionalization philosophies of the 1960s and 1970s (Powell and Hecimovic 1981; NYS OMRDD 1984; Cohen and Warren 1985). Many states have funded and developed respite services since the late 1960s. In New York State, funding for respite care has been available since 1974. In addition to OMRDD (Office of Mental Retardation and Developmental Disabilities), the Developmental Disabilities Act funds programs for respite care.

In New York City, more than a dozen respite programs exist to address the needs of families with mentally retarded or developmentally disabled (MRDD) children or adults. These MRDD respite care services are generally separate from the services for elderly or physically disabled persons. One exception is an overnight respite program located at a camp for blind persons and their families offered by VISIONS/Services for the Blind and Visually Impaired, a New York City-based agency. This overnight respite program at Vacation Camp for the Blind, located in Spring Valley,

New York, addresses the needs of families and blind developmentally disabled or multiply handicapped adults living at home (Weber 1991).

Published descriptions of respite care services in the United States for the elderly population and their family caregivers were first described in the mid-1970s (Pieper and Grundy 1977). Since then numerous demonstration projects and programs for the elderly population and their family caregivers have flourished (Tucker et al. 1980; Foundation for Long-Term Care 1985; Isett 1984; Scharlach and Frenzel 1985; NYS Department of Social Services 1985; Miller et al. 1986; Pennsylvania Department of Aging 1986). More than 15 respite care programs in New York City address the needs of families with elderly dependent relatives. In 1979, the New York State legislature passed the Community Services for the Elderly Act, which specifies respite care as a fundable service. Institutional respite care in nursing homes was funded by the state as a demonstration project in 1981. Also in 1981, the New York State legislature passed a respite care demonstration bill to fund free-standing and designated apartment-type overnight respite centers for elderly people. The demonstration has been extended, passed and refunded every year. In 1986 in New York State, the Extended In-Home Services for the Elderly Program (EISEP) was developed and funded to assist non-Medicaid eligible elderly persons with in-home care, including respite as a reimbursable service.

The current models of respite care functioning in New York State include:

- in-home respite care where a temporary care provider replaces the caregiver in the dependent person's home for a specified length of time
- institutional respite care providing temporary care overnight in an adult home, nursing home, camps or other residential facilities
- respite care cooperatives where caregivers provide care for one another's relatives
- respite centers usually with one or more apartments, or rooms with a small total bed capacity, providing overnight respite care exclusively, in a small home-like setting
- respite foster care where the dependent person lives temporarily in someone else's private home or apartment

Each of the models offered has advantages and disadvantages. The option most preferred is in-home respite care where the temporary caregiver moves into the home of the dependent person (Cohen and Warren 1985;

Weber 1986). However, respite care services are limited and families will often accept whatever services are available once they are made aware of them. Respite care is becoming a better known, more popular and expanding service. One reason is the media attention to the stresses on families of caregiving, the research addressing the stresses of caregiving, the growing awareness of Alzheimer's disease and its effect on families and a growing attitude in the workplace that supports families in accepting assistance when they are overburdened. State governments and health care insurers are encouraging any efforts that reduce demand for expensive nursing home care or paid home care workers for elderly persons. Respite care to support family caregiving is championed as a less costly service.

Evaluations of overnight institutional respite programs have indicated that there is, in some cases, an increased use of nursing home placement after a respite care stay (Foundation for Long-Term Care 1985). Documented in a Veterans Administration nursing home respite program in California, there were higher than normal admission rates within a month of a nursing home respite stay (Scharlach and Frenzel 1985). Explanations offered were based on feelings expressed by families that allowed them to more readily accept permanent nursing home placement, including their general surprise at the good quality of care and pleasant atmosphere, much better than what they had expected from a nursing home; a realization by families of the stress they were feeling and the toll it took as well as the exhaustion they allowed themselves to experience once the dependent person was not under their care which enabled them to give more consideration to how the caregiving impacted on their own well-being; and ability to overcome a sense of dread, fear and guilt over an institutional stay for their relative.

It is often the caregivers of persons who are the most difficult to care for or manage mentally or physically who have the fewest options for respite care but often need it the most. Generally, dependent persons with Alzheimer's disease, elderly physically disabled persons and multiply handicapped adults are served by the fewest number of programs (NYS OMRDD 1984; New York Association for the Blind 1984). In New York City, programs exist to serve these populations, but the needs far outweigh the current resources and knowledge among families of what does exist is limited.

Respite care services are clearly gaining attention as a service to families. Four books and two dissertations on respite care are available (Powell and Hecimovic 1981; Halpern 1981; Kayser 1984; Cohen and Warren 1985; Salisbury and Intagliata 1986; Montgomery and Prothero 1986).

GENERIC VS. SPECIALIZED SERVICES

Respite care programs have developed in a patchwork fashion—fragmented, funded inadequately, or funded with monies that are not secure from year to year. In addition, program development of respite care services has occurred within established networks of service. For the aging, respite care is often a program added to an already existing array of services sponsored by an organization serving frail elderly persons and their families. It may only be offered in the form easiest for the agency to implement. Respite care for the disabled population and their families often follows the establishment of services for a specific disability group, such as occurred for the MRDD population and the population with cerebral palsy where respite services are offered by the local UCP (United Cerebral Palsy) agency.

In New York City, as previously mentioned, there is only one agency for the blind that offers respite as an identifiable service. Most blind and severely visually impaired persons are independent and manage without the need for daily caregiving. However, the blind and visually impaired population is primarily elderly and vision problems are often associated with other health problems as the individuals grow older (Weber 1991). Another rapidly growing group are those blind persons with severe multiple disabilities developed at birth or at an early age. With the general growth of the elderly population, a growth in the number of school age children and medical advances that save the lives of babies born with severe multiple disabilities, individuals with vision impairments among both young and older ages are increasing. Based on a conservative estimate of 3 percent of the general population being legally blind or severely visually impaired, in New York City an estimated 240,000 persons have vision so limited that they are unable to read print even with glasses. Some individuals would be able to read regular or large print with special lighting, magnifiers or "low vision" lenses which would utilize their residual or remaining vision.

Legal blindness is the most severe vision impairment category and includes persons whose corrected vision in the better eye is 20/200 or worse, or those persons with less than 20 percent of their field of vision in both eyes. Using an estimate of 10 to 15 percent of the elderly population being legally blind or severely visually impaired, this would mean that there are approximately 130,000 to 150,000 elderly (60+) blind or severely visually impaired persons. Approximately 15,000 to 25,000 of these elderly blind or visually impaired persons are black, hispanic or Asian. These figures are growing dramatically in absolute numbers and as percentages of the total population, as the population of New York City ages, as minority group representation increases through immigration and longer life spans and as flight of the white population from the city continues. Only a small fraction of this legally blind and severely visually impaired population is currently being served by the blindness network of private, nonprofit and government organizations.

Historically, in the United States beginning in the 1800s, disabled people were segregated into special schools and workshops. The public's attitudes toward disabled people wavered between reverence, fear, pity, discomfort, revulsion and idolization. These reactions describe a common feeling that disabled people are different, sometimes "super" good, sometimes "super" evil, but always different. Among disabled people as a group, blind people were separated out for special services and attention. "Aid to the Blind" was a separate financial category and the State Commission for the Blind, responsible for rehabilitation and training, was often distinct from the Office of Vocational Rehabilitation, which served other disability groups. Efforts to politically unite disabled people in the 1970s emerged when legislation to prohibit discrimination on the basis of handicap was introduced. When the Rehabilitation Act of 1973 was passed a victory was won but separations among the various groups of, and advocates for, persons with disabilities continued. The passage of the Americans with Disabilities Act of 1990, which further prohibits discrimination was successful in part because of the coalitions built between disability groups and advocates for all persons with disabilities.

The concept of "mainstreaming" gained popularity as handicapped children and their families fought for the right to have public school education as a choice in addition to "special" schools or classes for handicapped children. As with the education of black children, at times separate meant unequal, of poorer quality or with fewer opportunities that would enable handicapped children to function socially or in employment situations alongside their sighted peers. The concept of mainstreaming expanded and is now used to describe any situation where handicapped and non-handicapped individuals are served together. However, practical experience has shown that just opening a door, offering an opportunity or an experience together is not necessarily enough. Sensitization, staff and teacher training, support and teaching the disabled child or adult the communication skills and adaptations necessary to function as independently as possible and overcome the particular obstacles posed by their disability, are all necessary conditions for mainstreaming or integrated services to be successful for both disabled and nondisabled participants. The earliest experiences of some handicapped children in regular classes was ridicule, ostracizing, academic failure and inability to compete or be as successful as their sighted or nondisabled peers. The schools and training programs learned that they also had to offer "special" teachers who could teach the specialized skills needed, such as braille for blind children, and provide the resources and equipment that would enable handicapped students to succeed with and take advantage of all the opportunities available to their nondisabled peers. However, problems in fully implementing this approach still exist; one example is the increasing illiteracy problem of blind children and young adults who have not been properly taught, or who have not mastered braille or other reading and communication methods (Spungin 1991).

RESPITE CARE SERVICES FOR THE BLIND AND THEIR FAMILIES

Respite care services are in their infancy. Policy choices are necessary in determining how to best develop and expand them. What should the service delivery system be? Should services be provided by an array of service agencies specialized to serve a particular disability group? Should services be provided by generic social service agencies who try to meet the needs of all families caring for a dependent individual regardless of age or the condition causing the dependency? Should respite services be offered by agencies serving the elderly, youth and children, often leaving persons in their middle years without appropriate services? In fact, choices have been made and are represented by the mixture of respite care services that do exist and are targeted by disability, by age (those specifically geared to older persons, children and young adults), and respite programs that try to address the needs of every family with a dependent person regardless of age or the cause of the dependent status. Since respite services are limited and often based on the availability of funding for one model over another, consumer preferences have not been the most influential factor in the development of many programs.

It is the authors' belief that the system to strive for is one that provides the most respite care choices for family caregivers and dependent persons because each family's situation is unique and their preferences are so individual. It is important to explore and document the preferences of user groups when choices do exist and to research the satisfaction and effectiveness of the various models of respite care in reducing stress and enhancing the sense of support felt by the caregiver and the care receiver in the family (Miller and Goldman 1988). There is still little known about the experiences of respite care from the perspective of the dependent person, or of their preferences among the various types of respite care services. One reason for this lack of information stems from a dilemma created by the various definitions identifying the client for respite care service. Some programs clearly reach out to caregivers as the client since the respite care is provided to give them relief. Some programs define the caregiver and the dependent person as the client, and following this definition of the family as the client, both are surveyed as to their satisfaction with the respite care service (Isett 1984; Pennsylvania Department of Aging 1986).

One survey conducted by Weber (1986) explored the knowledge and preference for respite care of 89 visually impaired elderly participants in an older adult center program at an agency for the blind. Out of the total membership of 289 blind participants, 89 older blind people lived with a relative and were mailed a large print questionnaire to fill out (if they had enough usable vision to complete it themselves, or given the choice to fill it out with a volunteer at the center). In all, 68 people completed the questionnaire (a 77.5 percent return rate). The findings, clearly only suggestive, indicated that while this group of older blind persons perceived respite care as a needed service for themselves and their families, most did not know what respite care was or that it existed as a service prior to getting the questionnaire, and if given a choice, the majority preferred the in-home respite care model even though they regularly attended the day center program at the agency. Most also stated they would consider staying at the agency's adult residence for overnight respite care if they needed it but could not get in-home services.

There is no clear evidence available to indicate whether or not all blind and visually impaired persons who need and request it are being served by respite care services for the general elderly or the general disabled population. Most programs, as part of their intake, do identify sensory and physical disabilities of the dependent person and in some research people with vision problems have been shown to be included among programs generally targeted for the elderly population. In an informal New York City survey (Weber 1986), most respite programs reported having served one or more visually impaired persons. It is not known how well the special needs of the blind or visually impaired person were met in the generic programs.

Blind and visually impaired persons and their families need access to respite care services. Agencies serving blind persons can add respite care as part of the array of services already provided such as camp programs, adult day centers, senior activity programs, youth programs and residential facilities. Respite care programs targeted to elderly and disabled populations can include blind or visually impaired persons in their regular services. Every state and most major cities or metropolitan areas have agencies serving blind persons who will help a local agency for the elderly or disabled adapt their services to best meet the needs of blind persons.

VISIONS/Services for the Blind and Visually Impaired in New York City uses its Vacation Camp for the Blind as a respite service site. Able to meet the needs of families where at least one member is blind or visually impaired, the camp offers year-round, flexible access to overnight respite care on weekends and during summer sessions. Families contribute toward the cost based on a self-assessed ability to pay. Participants using the site for respite pay the same amount as participants using the site as an overnight vacation camp. The camp is used for respite by elderly persons who are blind and their caregivers, as well as blind developmentally or multiply disabled adults and their families. Government funding for camp respite stays, and transportation to and from camp, is available only for those families who qualify under the guidelines of the New York State Office of Mental Retardation and Developmental Disabilities. This funding source covers the costs for most families with a blind, multiply handicapped family member who developed the disabilities prior to age 21. The camp respite program began when one caregiver approached the agency asking to use the site flexibly for temporary care. Currently, more than 60 families each year use Vacation Camp for the Blind as a respite care service.

> Mr. J, a 34-year-old, multiply impaired blind man with emotional and behavioral problems, lived with his mother, who was in her mid sixties. Mr. J had been attending summer sessions at Vacation Camp for the Blind for many years, giving his mother a break from providing daily care. His mother worked and had also been caring for her husband before he passed away after an extended illness. The mother had not been able to tell her son that his father had died, although he knew that his father was sick and that something was wrong. At his mother's request, over the course of the year, he attended all 8 scheduled 3-day weekends at Vacation Camp for the Blind. His mother finally had the strength to tell him his father had died. During the weekends, camp staff reminded him calmly and soothingly whenever he spoke about his father. He would pound the table and begin to cry. When he attended the 12-day summer camp session he said to staff, "Daddy is gone, won't come back," and that was the end of his emotional outbursts.

> Mrs. N, a blind mother in her eighties who was also a wheelchair user, lived with her sighted daughter. Mrs. N wanted to attend Vacation Camp for the Blind but refused to be separated from her daughter. The daughter, who gave full daily personal care to her mother needed a break. After speaking to staff, the camp agreed to accept them both as participants. During the day, camp staff provided relief care so that the daughter could rest and make use of the camp swimming pool and lake. Mrs. N was able to experience activities specifically adapted for participation by blind people and received personal care (toileting, dressing, etc.) as needed from camp staff. The two returned to camp for 3 summers until the mother passed away. After Mrs. N's death, her daughter told the staff that her stays at

Vacation Camp for the Blind were the bright spot in her year and that they had been her mother's greatest joy.

With the growth in the elderly blind population and increasing numbers of blind, multiply handicapped children and youth, respite care services are one answer to the pressures and strains on families.

REFERENCES

Brody, E.M. Women in the middle and family help to older people. *Gerontologist* 21(5):471-480, 1981.

Brubaker, T., ed. *Family Relationships in Later Life.* Beverly Hills: Sage Publications, 1983.

Census study reports 1 in 5 adults suffers from disability. *New York Times,* December 23, 1986, p. B7.

Cicerelli, V.G. *Helping Elderly Parents: The Role of Adult Children.* Boston: Cubaren House, 1981.

Cohen, S. and R. Warren. *Respite Care: Principles, Programs and Policies.* Austin TX: Pro-Ed, 1985.

Crews, John. E. Strategic planning and independent living for elders who are blind. *J. Visual Impairment Blindness,* February 1991, pp. 52-57.

Crossman, L., C. London and C. Barry. Older women caring for disabled spouses: a model for supportive services. *Gerontologist* 21(5):464-470, 1981.

Disability Statistics Abstract No. 3. U.S. Department of Education, National Institute on Disability and Rehabilitation Research (NIDRR), April 1992.

Fengler, A. and N. Goodrich. Wives of elderly disabled men: the hidden patients. *Gerontologist* 19(2):175-183, 1979.

Foundation for Long-Term Care. *Respite Care for the Frail Elderly, Monograph 1.* Albany, NY: The Center for the Study of Aging, 1985.

Frankfather, D. A., M. Smith and F. Caro. *Family Care of the Elderly.* Lexington, MA: D.C. Heath, 1981.

Halpern, P.L., Home-Based Respite Care and the Family Regenerative Power in Families with a Retarded Child. Unpublished doctoral dissertation, University of Maryland, 1981.

Horowitz, A. Sons and daughters as caregivers to older parents: differences in role performance and consequences. *Gerontologist* 25(6):612-617, 1985.

Horowitz, A. and R. Dobrof. *The Role of Families in Providing Care to the Frail and Chronically Ill Elderly Living in the Community.* New York: Brookdale Center on Aging of Hunter College, 1982.

Isett, R.D. *A Study of the Intercommunity Actions In-Home Respite Care Project.* Philadelphia: Mid-Atlantic Long-Term Care Gerontology Center, Temple University, December 1984.

Kaplan, D., A. Smith, R. Grobstein and S. Fischman. Family mediation of stress. *Social Work* 18:60-69, 1973.

Kayser, L.L. Women Caregivers: Stresses, Coping Mechanisms, and the Effectiveness of Respite Care. Unpublished doctoral dissertation, University of Maine, 1984.

Kingson, E., B. Hirshorn and J. Cornman. *Ties That Bind: Gerontological Society of America.* Cabin John, MD: Seven Locks Press, 1985.

Lowman, C. and C. Kirchner. Elderly blind and visually impaired persons: projected numbers in the year 2000. *J. Visual Impairment Blindness,* February 1979, pp. 69-73.

McCubbin, H. and S. Fegley, eds. *Stress and the Family,* Vols. 1 and 2. New York: Brunner/Mazel, 1983.

Miller, D.A. The sandwich generation: adult children of the aging. *Social Work* 26(5):419-423, 1981.

Miller, D. B. and L. Goldman. Perceptions of caregivers about special respite services for the elderly. *Gerontologist* 28(3):408-410, 1988.

Miller, D., N. Gulle, and F. McCue. The realities of respite for families, clients and sponsors. *Gerontologist* 26(5):467-470, 1986.

Montgomery, R. J. and J. Prothero, eds. *Developing Respite Services for the Elderly.* Seattle: University of Washington Press, 1986.

New York State Department of Social Services. Respite Demonstration Project Final Report. Albany, January 1985.

New York State Office of Mental Retardation and Developmental Disabilities. *Respite Services for Developmentally Disabled Individuals in New York State.* Albany, November 1984.

Orr, A., ed. *Vision and Aging: Crossroads for Service Delivery.* New York: American Foundation for the Blind, 1992.

Pennsylvania Department of Aging. *Determinants of Stress in Families Providing Care to Frail Elderly Relatives and the Effects of Receiving In-Home Respite Services,* Harrisburg, 1986.

Perlman, R., ed. *Family Home Care.* New York: Haworth Press, 1983.

Pieper, J. and L. Grundy. Respite care programs. *J. Gerontol. Nursing* 3(1):49, 1977.

Powell, T., B. Henessey and A. Hecimovic. *Respite Care for the Handicapped: Helping Individuals and Their Families.* Springfield, IL: Charles C Thomas, 1981.

Scharlach, A. and C. Frenzel. An evaluation of institution-based respite care. *Gerontologist* 25(2): 1985.

Selye, H. *Stress Without Distress.* J.B. Lippincott, 1974.

Silverstone, B. and H.K. Kandel. *You and Your Aging Parent.* New York: Pantheon Books, 1978.

Snyder, B. and K. Keefe. The unmet needs of family caregivers for frail disabled adults. *Social Work Health Care* 10(3):11-14, 1985.

Soldo, B. In-home services for the dependent elderly. *Research on Aging* 7(2):281-304, 1985.

Spungin, S.J. *Braille Literacy.* New York: American Foundation for the Blind, 1991.

Troll, L., S. Miller and R. Atchley. *Families in Later Life.* Belmont, CA: Wadsworth, 1979.

Tucker, D., J. Schmitter and T. Miklos. *Respite Care Survey and Report Findings.* Boston: Massachusetts Department of Mental Health, June 1980.

Weber, N.D. An Exploratory Survey of the Knowledge and Preferences of Visually Impaired Clients for Respite Services: A Supervisor/Student Project. Paper presented at the Annual New York State Association of Gerontological Educators (SAGE) Conference, 1986.

Weber, N.D., ed. *Vision and Aging: Issues in Social Work Practice.* Binghamton, NY: Haworth Press, 1991.

Issues in Respite Care

8

Programmatic and Caregiver Barriers to Respite Care*

Virginia W. Barrett, DrPH

Respite care refers to the whole variety of services offered to impaired elderly and their families, including adult day care (ADC). The number of ADC centers has grown rapidly, from a small number in the early 1970s to more than 2100 identified by the National Adult Day Care (NADC) census in 1989. According to this census, the number of ADC centers will need to continue to grow in the future to meet the needs of an increasing number of elderly who desire to remain in the community, but who require care and supervision to do so. The importance of this service and its need for expansion appear clear and yet many of these programs report difficulty maintaining the census required to meet the requirements of their funding agencies. In addition, studies have shown that ADC is not markedly effective in delaying institutional placement, in spite of the belief that it is an alternative care modality.

This chapter addresses possible barriers to respite day care services for the mentally impaired elderly that may account for census problems and difficulties in providing care. Barriers can originate from a variety of sources including the program itself, the client and the family. The content of this chapter draws on respite and other adult day care literature, a small 1991 survey of 14 ADC programs in two states and observa-

* The author acknowledges the support of the Columbia University Alzheimer's Disease Research Center—Research, Training and Information Transfer Core Project for this chapter, parts of which appear in their manuscript, "Respite Care: Problems of Mismatch."

tions made by this author during a 1986-87 study of disturbing behavior in mentally impaired elderly attending ADC.

On the program level, there appears to be a disparity between client needs and respite day care service provision, and a tendency to try to fit need to service rather than service to need. Prior to establishing a respite program, it is necessary to conduct a thorough, comprehensive needs assessment of the potential client population, but this is an infrequent practice. In situations where needs assessments are done, they may not be in accordance with guidelines appropriate to the service area. The majority of programs, for example, are located in metropolitan areas where potential clients may be from cultural backgrounds and family compositions that are quite different from those seen in more rural areas. When state guidelines for day care program development and needs assessment are generalized in ways that ignore environmental and cultural differences, the resulting organizational practices can negatively affect respite planning and program development.

The specific model of an ADC program can also affect service provision. Social model ADC, which primarily serves mentally impaired elderly, often rejects those with a diagnosis of Alzheimer's disease (Lawton 1989) and those who are physically ill and require medical care. Medical model day care often rejects applicants with obvious dementia. Although there may be a trend toward increasing the number of combined models in the future, the physically ill demented elderly are largely forgotten in this system at present; they constitute the nonusers (Weissert 1980).

Environmental barriers in ADC centers include a lack of availability of lifts, ramps and personnel to assist with transfer activities, leading to the exclusion of clients in wheelchairs (Mace and Rabins 1984), and an absence of spacious walking areas and security systems to prevent escape from the program area, leading to the exclusion of clients who wander.

The process by which a potential client of respite care is referred can also interfere with service provision. Some people, usually health professionals, making referrals for day care, are not always fully aware of the limitations of the services provided, or may use the referral as a way to disengage from further involvement with a "difficult" client. In addition, the people who are involved in making the referral are not necessarily those involved in supervising the transition to this type of care and therefore are not fully aware of the multifaceted activities and the sensitive approach required to make the transition a smooth one.

The respite program client, especially in the early stages of a dementing illness, may create barriers to service by refusing or being reluctant to attend the program. This refusal to attend is often associated with the client's not feeling comfortable with, or being fearful of the behaviors of the other clients, or being separated from the primary caregiver and the familiar home environment. The client who wanders or who is agitated may continually try to leave the center and reject program activities that require sitting for any period of time. These problems can often be avoided if, prior to attendance, a comprehensive home assessment has taken place. A history of past interests and activities should be determined as well as the nature of the client's current abilities or disabilities. This assessment should also include identifying situations that appear to trigger behavior changes. Trial visits to the program for increased periods of time and continual reassurance are required for a smooth transition to respite day care.

When the concept of respite service in the form of ADC is not properly presented to the family caregivers of an impaired elderly person, their response may become a barrier to program success. Despite the intention of respite services to assist families in caregiving they sometimes take over some of the activities previously provided by family members. When this occurs, the resulting change in the caregiving role can be threatening, especially if the family caregiver is greatly immersed in the role. Respite services may be interpreted by the caregiver as a negative critique of the care previously provided and a threat to their role continuity in the family. It may challenge the caregiver's self-esteem, religious and moral values, beliefs about care equity or caring for the parent who cared for them in childhood, and caregiver modeling, or setting an example for the next generation (Lawton et al. 1989).

The caregiver may feel loss of control and loss of secondary benefits of the caregiving role, such as praise from others for their sacrifices. They may also feel that decreasing the time for caregiving activity means that they have to give time to other more troublesome activities that could previously have been avoided, such as getting a job, socializing, taking care of themselves, or attending to other more difficult relationships or responsibilities. Moritz and co-workers (1987) report that once relieved of the caregiving role, spouse caregivers may experience symptoms of dysphoric mood and decreased participation in certain social and leisure activities. Caregivers with this reaction may be uninterested in the opportunity provided by respite to increase participation in activities that caregiving has prevented.

Examples of situations in which the caregiving role provides secondary gains are numerous. One program reported the case of a middle-aged caregiver who provided years of care to his demented mother, despite her physical abuse of him during his childhood and verbal abuse in his adult years. His continuing need for her approval and love was the driving force behind his assuming responsibility for her care, even though she no longer recognized him.

Another program described a family caregiver with marital difficulties who cared for her demented mother. When her husband requested that they engage in marital counseling to try to resolve their difficulties, she responded by moving into her mother's apartment with the explanation that her mother's need of her time outweighed his.

In the situations described above, the secondary gains to the caregivers, however dysfunctional the circumstances, outweighed the benefits that respite services could have provided. Caregivers frequently need to be assured that their role is not being usurped and to be urged to seek counseling. Family caregivers may also be so overwhelmed by their caregiving role that respite care seems to give them an additional burden rather than relief from it. The burden they feel in caregiving is at least familiar, whereas initially the demands that come with involvement in the program are not. These demands include getting the client ready to go to the program at a specific time, having to telephone the program director if there is any change in plan, making sure that the client has everything he needs for the day (medications, extra clothes, incontinence pads, etc.), filling out forms, getting the client's physician to send reports to the program, attending support groups and getting someone to stay with the client while they are attending the meetings, and finally, being at the day care center to collect the client at a specific time or being at home to wait for the client to be delivered by a transportation service at a specific time. All of these changes in routine may be interpreted as extra work, and not worth the effort.

In any event, stressed family caregivers usually feel that their situation is unique and that stress produced by change in daily activity is greater than could be imagined by others. Poor attendance at caregiver support groups may largely be due to this feeling of unique burden that is painful to share and perceived by the caregiver as impossible for others to fully understand. It is not uncommon for families providing care to demented elderly to experience mental and physical symptoms of stress such as anxiety and agitation, loss of patience, insomnia and sleep disruption, pessimism, palpitations, loss of appetite, and digestive problems, all of which contribute to feelings of isolation and immobility.

Family caregivers may also create barriers to service provision when they have difficulty accepting that their elder is impaired to the extent that respite service is needed. The first visit by the family member to a respite day care program is traumatic, even when the family has been forewarned. At the time of the first visit they may still be denying the illness and severity of symptoms and they are not familiar with the impairments of the other clients attending the program. Frequently expressed responses of caregivers to first seeing the program's clients gathered in a room include: "My mother isn't that bad"; "I'm not sure this is the right place for her"; "She wouldn't have anything in common with these people"; "Who would she talk to?" and "She's so used to me taking care of her that she'd never let others do it."

Even when the client adjusts to the program, family caregivers respond with a variety of emotions ranging from relief to guilt to expressions of long-standing anger displaced onto staff. The best developed plans for care of a client can be sabotaged by family caregivers if negative feelings and other problems are not identified and dealt with by the service providers from the beginning.

Family caregivers who express discontent with day respite services often speak about the way the program fails to meet their specific needs in caring for their elders. Areas of expressed discontent with the program include the time of operation, which may conflict with the hours when they need relief from caregiving responsibilities to hold a job; services that the program doesn't provide, such as physical therapy, distribution of medication, special dietary regimes, and transportation to and from the program. Just as the needs of each client and family are unique, the programs themselves also differ from one another in terms of services provided and add to the possibilities of conflict between need and service provision.

The management of client behaviors that are disturbing to others is another factor seen in programs providing care to the demented elderly and may result in conflict between families and staff. Behavior changes exhibited by the client that are disturbing to the family are not necessarily the ones that are disturbing to the staff of the respite day care program. Wandering, for example, may be easily controlled by the family after additional locks are put on doors in the house. However, at the day care center, wandering may be more of a safety hazard as well as a liability to the program if fire regulations prohibit the locking of doors and financial constraints prohibit the installation of warning devices. Some centers, according to the Survey of Day Care for Demented Adults, report that they reject clients with severely disruptive behaviors that are thought to be "inappropriate for day care" in spite of the fact that these behaviors are symptomatic of the disease affecting most of the clients. Most surveyed programs said they would not accept clients with a history of violent behavior and many had had to discharge clients for unmanageable behaviors. Incontinence was tolerated to varying degrees by different centers. As previously stated, there was a wide variety of types and tolerance of disturbing behaviors reported. There was also no relationship

between discharges due to disturbing behavior and the number of demented clients attending the program. Since there is a tendency toward
more aggressive and wandering behavior with the more severely demented (Burns et al. 1990), services may be more apt to be discontinued
when the family needs them the most.

The findings of this author's 1986-87 study (Barrett 1988) of disturbing behavior in a population of mentally impaired elderly who attended
two ADC programs suggested that client behaviors, particularly 12 identified as threatening to the interpersonal relationship between client and
primary family caregiver, had the greatest associations with measures of
family caregiver burden and institutional planning. These included:
suspiciousness, being ungrateful, coldness toward others, rejecting others, complaining, reassurance seeking, repetitive questioning, demanding, arguing, manipulation, clinging and refusing to attend day care. By
contrast, the day care staff found it more stressful to handle behaviors that
threatened staffing patterns, legal considerations and job satisfaction.

The primary goal of respite care is to provide services to the
impaired individual and relief to the family caregiver, thereby postponing
or preventing premature or unnecessary institutionalization. Presumably
the client should be able to remain on an ADC program providing a lack
of acute illness, family problems, moving out of the program's catchment
area, or death. But there appear to be other reasons or barriers to service
that account for clients who are in need of services but who do not attend.
Most of these are associated with a change in the client's behavior or the
caregiver's needs that cannot be accommodated by the ADC program. As
concluded by Mace and Rabins (1984), transfer to a nursing home cannot
be used to describe a causal relationship between day care and nursing
home placement rates. Each situation is unique and the reasons for
discontinuation of day care services are multifaceted.

Because the existing literature on reasons for service discontinuation and client discharge from respite care is limited, a brief survey was
conducted by this author in 1991 of 14 day care center directors of
programs offering respite services to mentally impaired elderly. Respondents were asked to compare demographic, family and living arrangements, health status and service use, independence in activities of daily
living, memory impairment and behavioral characteristics of clients discharged from the program in the past year with those currently attending.

The findings of this survey showed that the centers had a range of
12 to 89 clients and a range of 0 to 48 discharges over the past year. As
expected, the programs varied in staff composition and services provided.
Differences in age, gender, income and education between center clients
were not remarkable. Ethnic composition showed differences reflecting

the communities served by the programs and there was a disproportion-
ate percentage of blacks, hispanics and other nonwhites among the clients
discharged. The family caregivers were mainly spouses and daughters, as
expected for this group of impaired elderly, but in the centers where there
were more nonwhites, the caregivers were more often paid home aides.
The discharged clients were reported to be at least as cognitively impaired
and physically frail as those currently attending the programs, and most
reported that these clients required more personal care assistance and
more supervision in activities of daily living. There was generally no
difference in the living arrangements of discharged clients.

The directors at each of the adult day care programs were also asked
why their clients were discharged in the past year. Presented with a list of
36 possible reasons for discharge, other than nursing home placement,
each was asked to indicate which one described their discharged clientele,
and which were primary or secondary causes. The reasons stated represented many problems surrounding care of the mentally impaired elderly
in the community, and covered a variety of circumstances. The results
indicated that the reasons for discharge are complex and are rarely
attributable to one cause. They may emanate from the limitations of the
program services available, changes in client health status, changes in
client behaviors, family problems, and discontent with services, among
other possibilities.

From mild to moderate to severe stages of dementing illness, the
need for services change, and unless the changing needs are identified
and services tailored to meet them, respite day care cannot function as
an alternative to institutionalization or a caregiving partner to family
members.

Respite care for the mentally impaired elderly is not a "miracle
intervention" (Lawton et al. 1989), and the success and failures of one
program type cannot be generalized to others (Montgomery and Prothero 1986). Although the focus of this chapter has been on the barriers
to optimal respite day care services, the implications for areas of improvement are evident. It appears that in the enthusiastic effort to develop
increased numbers of programs in this country, attention to improving
their quality through fitting service to need has been somewhat over-
looked. As reported by Wallace (1990), in looking at availability, accessibility and acceptability in community-based long-term care, caregivers
view respite care as "the most needed unavailable service."

Rather than putting our efforts toward increasing the numbers of
ADC centers, it would appear that a practical approach to program
development is needed that focuses on client and family caregiver needs
in the existing adult day care centers, rather than the bureaucratic and

managerial needs of the service agencies. Suggested program elements include: (1a) careful assessment of the population to be served prior to program development, with input from families in the geographic area to be served, and (1b) in-home assessments of every applicant with attention to functional ability, behaviors, interests and family dynamics; (2) more flexible admission criteria which do not exclude clients because of diagnosis, multiple impairments, behaviors, language spoken, or financial status; (3) a multidisciplinary team approach to environmental planning and case management, and when possible, staff composition representative of the cultural backgrounds of the clients; (4) a wider range of services including personal care, hours that meet the needs of the working family caregivers, and education and support programs for family members; (5) a clear agreement with families regarding their role and what they can expect in the way of support; (6) an active position for ADC in the continuum of care which helps to make transitions to acute care and long-stay situations occur with ease; (7) ongoing comprehensive program evaluation activities and client assessments for the purpose of identifying change in clients in terms of function and behavior, and need for program change; and (8) continuation of research activities that focus specifically on the effect of respite day care on nursing home postponement and the quality of life of the client and caregiver. Above all, client- and family-centered policy is needed in respite day care that is committed to the ideal that the program exists to serve the client and family, regardless of changes in client behaviors. The focus on preventing premature institutional placement should not preclude attention to the client's and caregiver's quality of life. Provision of care to mentally frail elderly is an ever-changing process and the challenge it presents needs to be met in an atmosphere that welcomes flexible interventions and creative programming.

REFERENCES

Barrett, V.W. Disturbing Behavior in Mentally Impaired Elderly. Unpublished doctoral dissertation, Columbia University School of Public Health, New York, 1988.

Burns, A., R. Jacoby and R. Levy. Behavioral abnormalities and psychiatric symptoms in Alzheimer's disease: preliminary findings. *Int. Psychogeriatrics* 2(1):25-36, 1990.

Caserta, M.S., et al. Caregivers to dementia patients: the utilization of community services. *Gerontologist* 27(2):209-214, 1987.

Cohen, S. and R.D. Warren. *Respite Care: Principles, Programs and Policies.* Austin, TX: Pro-Ed, 1985.

Foundation for Long-Term Care. *Respite Care for the Frail Elderly.* Albany, NY: The Center for the Study of Aging, 1983.

Lawton, M.P., E. Brody and A. Saperstein. Respite care for Alzheimer's families: research findings and their relevance to providers. *Am. J. Alzheimer's Care,* November/December 1989, pp.3-38.

Mace, N.L. and P.V. Rabins. *A Survey of Day Care for the Demented Adult in the United States.* Department of Psychiatry and Behavioral Sciences, Johns Hopkins University School of Medicine, National Council on the Aging, December 1984.

Montgomery, R.J.V. and J. Prothero, eds., *Developing Respite Services for the Elderly.* Seattle: University of Washington Press, 1986.

Moritz, D.J., S.V. Kasl and L.F. Berkman. The health impact of living with a cognitively impaired elderly spouse: depressive symptoms and social functioning *J. Gerontol.* 44(1):S17-S27, 1989.

Petry, S., et al. Personality alterations in dementia of the Alzheimer's type. *Arch. Neurol.* 45:1187-1190, 1988.

Wallace, S.P. The no-care zone: availability, accessibility, and acceptability in community-based long-term care. *Gerontologist* 30(2):254-261, 1990.

Weissert. W., et al. Effects and costs of day care services for the chronically ill: a randomized experiment. *Medical Care* 18(6):567-584, 1980.

Winogrod, I.R., et al. The relationship of caregiver burden and morale to Alzheimer's disease patient function in a therapeutic setting, *Gerontologist* 27(3):336-339, 1987.

Zarit, S.H., K.E. Reeves and J. Bach-Peterson. Relatives of the impaired elderly: correlates of feelings of burden. *Gerontologist* 20(6):649-655, 1980.

9

Financial, Medical, Personal and Social Barriers to Respite Care

Peter V. Rabins, MD

The undesirable physical effects of caregiving for chronically ill individuals were first described a quarter of a century ago by Sanford (1975) and Grad and Sainsbury (1963) in Great Britain. In the late 1970s, the difficulties experienced caregivers of cognitively impaired individuals was also documented by a number of authors (Lezak 1978; Zarit 1980) and launched a broad field of descriptive intervention research (Malonebeach 1991). These studies demonstrate that caregivers of the chronically ill have higher rates of psychological distress (anger, depression, guilt) and physical fatigue, use more tranquilizers and make more doctor visits than matched non-caregivers (see, for example, George and Gwyther, 1986).

Respite services—services that allow those that provide care to the ill personal time away from the activity—are one of the proposed solutions for this range of undesired effects. A wide variety of services fit under this umbrella. They include: in-home aide and nursing services; day treatment center programs; brief nursing home placement services; and informal help from friends and family. Surprisingly, even though the need for respite is high, these services have not been utilized by many of the people who appear to need them. Some services have failed because of lack of economic viability and others have closed because of lack of use. It is the experience of many clinicians and caregiver support groups that many individuals who might benefit from the service do not want to use it.

Empirical studies (Lawton 1989) demonstrate a similar finding. Equally surprising is that many individuals who eventually do use respite services do so long after the time that they need it. Indeed, a common clinical impression is that respite services are often used when it is "too late" and a permanent change in residence such as institutionalization is already inevitable.

What might be the sources of this resistance to service use? Unfortunately, we have little empirical data or research to help us answer this question. Several plausible reasons suggest themselves.

FINANCIAL BARRIERS

Undoubtedly, financial considerations affect the decision to use respite services. Professional in-home care can range from $5.00 to $12.00 per hour, and adult day care centers cost $40.00 to $60.00 per day on average. Some services are able to give financial help or have sliding-scale fee schedules, but the uncertainty about how long a service might be used, the limited and fixed incomes of many older persons and the limitation of financial resources themselves are often barriers.

DISEASE BARRIERS

A second set of barriers relates to the types of emotional and behavioral difficulties experienced by the ill person. Individuals with dementia may be fearful about "strangers" and may misinterpret their motives. It is not uncommon for a patient to "fire" a paid helper, a behavior many care providers and family members find difficult or impossible to override or ignore. Some patients are reluctant to leave the house or to go to strange places. Many patient behaviors become so difficult that they may drive the respite worker from the home or render the patient unmanageable at a respite site. Also, the physical care needs of patients may be too severe. For example, some day centers are unable to manage the incontinent (Mace and Rabins 1984).

CAREGIVER ISSUES

Caregivers themselves may resist use of the services because they feel they "should be able to handle everything." To these individuals, asking for help, whether it be from family or friends, is the wrong thing to do. Such persons have often been hard-working and independent all their lives and appear to have psychological characteristics that prevent them from accepting help. Others feel that no one can do as good a job as they can and, indeed, sometimes they are right. Nonetheless, in the long run, their refusal to accept help may be detrimental both to them and to the patient if something untoward happens to the caregiver.

We sometimes see this refusal to accept services as "neurotic," as a manifestation of resistance or as evidence of denial. Undoubtedly, each of these mechanisms does influence the choice by some caregivers not to use respite. On the other hand, there is a heroic, admirable side to this behavior. It can also be seen as reflecting the central role that family obligations have in shaping behavior. Appreciating this cultural context and seeing its positive as well as its negative aspects may help the family eventually to accept respite services.

COMMUNITY AND SOCIAL ISSUES

At a community level, the resistance to respite can be seen as arising from several sources. The idea that accepting outside help is undesirable is a shared cultural value and needs to be considered at that level. Another broad societal issue is the lack of understanding about chronic illness and its prevalence. Many elements of the American medical system—its emphasis on individual practitioners, the acute general hospital, the Medicare payment system and the low regard in which nursing homes are held—reflect a lack of awareness and even a denial that chronic illness is common and becoming increasingly prevalent. This results in both a lack of support and a lack of interest in services such as respite.

DISCUSSION AND IMPLICATIONS

The first question that must be addressed is whether the respite care model, as currently conceptualized, is failing because the need for respite services is minimal, whether there is no need because the current system is poorly conceptualized or because various barriers prevent the current model's implementation. Many surveys of caregivers who present to support groups or Alzheimer's disease research centers find that families say the need for respite is great. While these are not population-based samples, the results suggest that caregivers *believe* that more respite care is needed. Therefore, it is more likely that the current models of respite care are designed in such a way that they do not meet needs and that the barriers to their implementation and acceptance prevents utilization. Since either of these alternatives is possible, it does not make sense to focus only on the barriers. The possibility that the current respite conceptualization is wrong needs further careful thought. Nonetheless, a consideration of the barriers to implementation suggests several possible approaches to overcoming the lack of utilization of respite services:

1. The barriers to acceptance of respite need to be addressed individually; most likely they vary from site to site and family to family.
2. New models of respite need to be considered. While the range of services—in-home, day care and brief nursing home stay—is broad, different combinations of these or different forms of respite may need to be developed to overcome barriers of acceptance and increase the likelihood of implementation. Financial supports, visiting nurse controlled beds (as used in Great Britain) and better use of volunteers are among the possibilities.
3. Referral services need to be better developed. Better use of formal (physician, social service agency, research clinic) and nonformal (churches, radio and TV spots, newspaper articles, support groups, Alzheimer's Association chapters) referral sources might increase utilization.
4. Current services may be more accepted if they are better integrated. This would make them more flexible as well. For example, services combining in-home and day care or day care and nursing home respite might benefit certain individuals. Integrating agencies or having single agencies with more direct contact with respite services would include in-home health services, day care and brief inpatient stays. All of these modalities might increase utilization if service integration was more acceptable.

REFERENCES

George, L.K. and L.P. Gwyther. Caregiver well-being: a multidimensional examination of family caregivers of demented adults. *Gerontologist* 26:253-259, 1986.

Grad, P. and P. Sainsbury. Mental illness and the family. *Lancet* 1:544-577, 1963.

Lawton, M.P., E. Brody and A. Saperstein. Respite care for Alzheimer's families: research findings and their relevance to providers. *Am. J. Alzheimer's Care* November/December, 1989, pp. 31-38.

Lezak, M.D. Living with the characterologically altered brain injured patient. *J. Clin. Psychiatry* 39 592-598, 1978.

Mace, N.L., P.V. Rabins. *A Survey of Day Care for the Demented Adult in the United States.* Washington, DC: National Council on Aging, 1984.

Malonebeach, E.E. and S.H. Zaret. Current research issues in caregiving to the elderly. *Int. J. Aging Human Development* 32:103-114, 1991.

Sanford, J. Tolerance of disability in elderly dependents by supports at home: its significance for hospital practice. *Br. Med. J.* 3:471-473, 1975.

Zarit, S.H., K.E. Reever and J. Bach-Peterson. Relatives of the impaired elderly: correlates of feelings of burden. *Gerontologist* 20:649-655, 1980.

10

Changing Needs
in Adult Day Care

Katherine Manning, BS, RN

In 1973 the Community Centers for Mental Health sponsored a social recreation program for senior citizens that offered activities and social services counseling on a limited basis—1 day per week. After 1 year this program expanded; run by a facilitator, it offered daily activities and was moved to its own barrier-free facility (an annex 200 feet from the main building). However, we discovered that ambulation problems, confusion and even cardiac impairments caused the frail elderly to withdraw from the recreation program (or to never attend it in the first place). We identified the need to assist those who were unable to utilize existing services because of physical, mental or cognitive disabilities. As a result, in December 1977, the Northern Valley Older Adult Day Center was developed. As a social day care program our services expanded to include transportation, nursing and nutritional services. Staff also increased to include a full-time director, an activities director, a nurse and a driver. The staff/client ratio grew to 1:5.

Today, the Northern Valley Older Adult Day Center provides day care to the frail elderly of sixteen communities in Bergen County, New Jersey. Our program is in operation from 8:30 a.m. to 4:30 p.m., Monday through Friday. Our day care program provides a safe, structured, therapeutic program for the elderly client and also provides respite for the caregiver. The services offered include: health supervision, crisis intervention, social services, individual and family counseling and pre-entry screening that includes consultation with the family. In addition to care of the frail elderly, we offer a monthly support group for the "sandwich generation" and weekly blood pressure, weight and pulse checks for all seniors in the community.

At the start, in 1977, Community Development funded 100 percent of this program. Over the years this source of funding dropped to 31 percent of the total budget. This is partly due to a decrease in actual dollar amounts from Community Development as well as increases in our budget. In the past we sought funding from the Division on Aging (Title III), but, unfortunately, we found that these funds were committed to other programs. While doing research for this chapter, I found in our files copies of letters to nongovernmental sources (i.e., foundations and companies) requesting funds; there were also many letters of regret.

In 1980 two concerns forced us to re-evaluate our day care program: (1) funding from traditional sources had decreased, and (2) clients who were part of the first phase of the Greystone Park Psychiatric Hospital deinstitutionalization initiative and who were participating in our Psychiatric Partial Care Program at the Community Centers for Mental Health were "aging out" and their needs were changing from purely psychiatric to social/medical care as well. The decision was made to redefine the adult day care program into a social/psychiatric partial care program. This enabled us to tap additional sources of income.

As the population ages and families are caring for their elderly family members longer at home, the caregiver is in need of assistance and respite. We have seen elderly people attending our program in a frailer and more physically disabled state than ever before.

The 1990 census figures for our 16-town catchment area indicated that there were 31,880 persons over the age of 60 and 2032 people over the age of 84. It is estimated that 5 percent of all people over the age of 60 in the United States are in need of long-term care. In our catchment area alone, this translates into 1600 persons over the age of 60 and 102 persons over the age of 84 who could be in need of long-term care.

Adult day care is an important component of the long-term care continuum. The spectrum of quality services that we provide to our clients enables them to remain at home for a longer period of time before they have to be placed in a nursing home. Recent evaluation of our program indicates that our clients' medical needs have changed and that we will be able to serve them better if we are designated as a medical day care facility and we are now applying to the state to be licensed as an adult day health care facility (ADHF). We have already taken steps to redesign the facility in order to comply with additional state requirements.

Our program is a warm, friendly home away from home where confused, frail elderly are not threatened or laughed at, but rather are treated with dignity and respect. They are free to remember and share their past with their peers. People in our program have done things they never did before in their 70 or 80 years of life—simple things that others might take for granted, such as going to a local museum, the theater, or even a restaurant. One of our 85-year-old clients had never gone to a restaurant until she went with our group. She also told us in a group discussion that one thing she always wanted to do was to go to a museum to see beautiful paintings. So, we all went and she truly enjoyed herself. We had made a dream come true.

Many times caregivers think their family member has lost touch with reality or has become incontinent when in fact this is not true, or at least not irreversibly so. In fact, after working with certain individuals we have found that very simple strategies can often overcome these problems. For example, a family may believe their elderly family member is incontinent when, in fact, the older person simply forgot to use the toilet or waited too long, and this caused the accident, not incontinence. Years ago our center did not admit clients who were incontinent. Now, however, with the advent of commercially available absorbent pads for adults, we admit these supposedly incontinent persons. With attention to toileting every few hours, we find that most participants are not incontinent while they are in our program.

Socialization with their peers seems to help elders to overcome their fears and sense of isolation. It is wonderful to watch a frightened, shy, elderly lady brighten up just because her peer has touched her hand or offered her a favorite seat. Medical monitoring and socialization are important outcomes of an adult day care program.

Respite for the primary caregiver is another major outcome of day care programs. Children of the elderly are able to work, care for their own children, and sometimes get a break for themselves. Our "Sandwich Generation Support Group" for caregivers is an important adjunct to our program. Here caregivers can share their hopes and fears, ask questions and hear others speak on various topics of concern to themselves and their elderly family member.

It is often the case that spouses, especially male spouses, have great difficulty in "letting go" of ongoing care for their partners. An example will illustrate this point. Mrs. Kelly had Alzheimer's disease and was cared for at home by her husband. They had three children, two daughters and a son who lived out of the area. The children were concerned but geographically unable to help their father take care of their mother. When they did visit, they would leave him a list of things he should do. (One daughter was a nurse, another a social worker.) During one visit home the children stopped by our center and discussed the situation. When I offered to come to their home, Mr. Kelly was reluctant to let me visit. However, his daughters had gone back home and I think he was lonely. I visited and interviewed him and his wife, but he did not want her to attend the program. I called him on a regular basis, and visited him again. After 2 months Mr. Kelly agreed to have his wife come 2 days a week, transporting her himself. He would come in the morning, stay for a cup of coffee, and in the afternoon he would talk for awhile. Within 3 months Mrs. Kelly was attending 5 days a week and Mr. Kelly was having his blood pressure and weight checked on a regular basis. His family and I would call each other when anything happened. He became very comfortable and reliant on the staff at the center. Mrs. Kelly attended the center 5 days a week for over a year. This is just one example of the type of family situations that we deal with every day. Not only does adult day care become a second home to the clients but in many cases it also becomes an extended home to the caregiver.

Clearly, adult day care is much more than a "baby sitting" service. The elderly people who attend day care are treated with the dignity and respect they deserve. The total effect on the elderly person's emotional and physical health is monumental.

This is a very promising time in adult day care; corporations are seeing the need for respite for their employees, legislators are aware of the high cost of long-term care and are talking about legislation for adult day care. Those involved in caregiving are excited to be part of this aspect of the continuum of long-term care.

WHAT IS ADULT DAY CARE AND WHAT SERVICES DOES IT PROVIDE?

Adult day care is an important component of the long-term care continuum. As mentioned before, the many different services that adult day care centers can offer allow elderly adults to live at home for a longer period of time before being placed in a nursing home.

Adult day care provides a safe, structured, therapeutic program for the elderly client and at the same time provides respite for the caregiver. The services offered include: health supervision, crises intervention, social services, individual and family counseling, pre-entry screening, transportation and nutritional services. A monthly "sandwich generation" support group and weekly blood pressure, weight and pulse checks for all seniors in the community are also provided.

WHAT BENEFITS ARE DERIVED BY CLIENTS AND CAREGIVERS FROM ADULT DAY CARE?

Adult day care provides a temporary home away from home where confused, frail elderly are treated with dignity and respect. We have found that socialization with peers seems to help the elderly to overcome the fear and isolation that so often accompany old age. Medical monitoring, socialization and respite are all important outcomes of a successful adult day care program. In a nation where more than 15 percent of all persons over the age of 60 are in need of some form of long-term care, society as a whole benefits from a compassionate, thoughtfully designed and implemented system of adult day care.

11

Financing Care
for the Chronically Ill:
The Respite Care Factor

Gerald Rosner, CLU, ChFC
and JoAnn Canning, RN, CLU, ChFC

The problem of providing acceptable care for the chronically ill is often strained by the collateral and sometimes conflicting expense of advances in available life-expanding technologies. Yet "caring should always take priority over curing for the most obvious of reasons: there is never any certainty that our illness can be cured or...death averted" (Eisenberg 1977). Most people with lengthy terminal illness will require at least some institutional care and all people with an illness will require some home care. It is in these areas that our society is most deficient; emphasis has been placed on curing over caring.

The same advances that have prolonged our lives so dramatically have given rise to increasing paid and unpaid costs of support for the chronically ill. This chapter will try to outline the financial resources that are available to these individuals. The respite care factor—cost and supply of resources for respite care—will be explored within the microcosm of New York City.

The quality of these lives—the caregiver and recipient—is unfairly diminished. As Callahan put it, our system of health care must "above all...be prepared to support and minister to people in their vulnerability to sickness and death, which can only be reduced, never vanquished. That is the one assurance we must have from our fellow human beings" (Callahan 1990).

CASE HISTORIES

Changes in functional status are due to a wide range of health conditions: arthritis, neurological problems, cancer and diabetes, to name a few. Over time most of these conditions are deteriorative and require increasing amounts of care. For illustrative purposes, the National Institutes of Health (1986) supplies factual data about one of these health conditions—amyotrophic lateral sclerosis (ALS).

- ALS is a disease of middle age.
- Half of all ALS patients diagnosed before age 50 live for more than 7 years after the diagnosis.
- Half of all ALS patients live 3 years or more after diagnosis; 20 percent live 5 years or more.
- Up to 10 percent live more than 10 years after diagnosis.

ALS rarely requires institutional care. The care required is defined by government and private insurance carriers as "custodial" care and is almost never a covered expense. As a result, the burden of caring for an ALS patient falls on family, friends and when it is affordable, a professional caregiver paid by the patient or the patient's family.

In a book called *This Far and No More*, A.H. Malcolm describes the case of a husband who watches his wife slowly weaken from the effects of ALS. He sees her gasp for breath, realizes the disease has reached her lungs and is torn between rushing her to a hospital or allowing her to die. The husband and wife had never discussed the use of heroic measures. She becomes unconscious and he becomes numb. Throughout the book there is passing mention of large expenses incurred, such as the need to sell a country house to pay for nurses and aides, but no specific figures are given, leaving the reader curious as to how, on one moderate salary, all of the attendant costs of a lengthy illness were covered by this family.

Oliver Sacks' celebrated book *Awakenings* discusses some twenty case histories of people with parkinsonism. Except for one fleeting mention of federal cutbacks, there is no reference to costs, which were undoubtedly horrendous. As well, there are no statistics in the prologues, epilogues or case histories on the price of maintaining these incapacitated people in an institution for periods of 25 years or more.

SOURCES OF FINANCING: MEDICARE COVERAGE

Skilled Care

Medicare will cover skilled nursing in a nursing home. However, no custodial care coverage is provided, nor is there any benefit paid for private duty nursing in hospitals. The following conditions must be satisfied before Medicare will help pay for inpatient care in a skilled nursing facility:

1. Hospitalization for at least 3 consecutive days.
2. Transfer to a skilled nursing facility (SNF) to receive care for the same conditions for which the patient had been hospitalized.
3. Physician certification that skilled nursing care is needed on a daily basis.
4. Entry into the SNF within 30 days after discharge from the hospital.
5. Written approval by a Medicare intermediary.

If all of these conditions are met, the maximum period of coverage is 100 days per benefit period. Again Medicare does not cover private duty nursing or custodial care in a skilled nursing facility.

Home Care

Medicare will pay for covered home health care services only when furnished by a participating home health care agency and only if all of the following conditions are met:

1. The care required includes intermittent skilled nursing care and physical or speech therapy.
2. The patient must be confined to the home.
3. A physician must certify that home health care is required under a plan designed by the doctor.
4. The home health care agency rendering the services has to be preapproved by Medicare.

No coverage is provided for general household services such as meal preparation, shopping or other domestic needs. The nursing care must be part-time, for example, up to 8 hours per day for up to 21 days. Drugs and transfusions are not covered.

Hospice Care

Under the Medicare hospice care provisions, respite coverage for both home and inpatient care is provided on a limited basis. A participating hospice is also permitted to provide appropriate custodial care, including homemaker services and counseling. The following conditions must be satisfied:

1. A doctor must determine that the patient is terminally ill.
2. The patient must elect hospice care.
3. The hospice must be preapproved.

Special benefits are provided for a maximum of two 90-day periods and one 30-day period. The benefit periods may be consecutive. If a beneficiary disenrolls during a benefit period, the remainder of the benefit period is lost by the individual, public agency, or private agency. Respite care may be delivered in the following types of settings: medical adult day care, social adult day care, residential skilled nursing care and residential other than skilled nursing and home care.

THE RESPITE CARE FACTOR

In the June 1990 *Respite Guide* issued by New York State Office for the Aging, policy is at odds with rhetoric. The conclusion reached is that although cost is often cited as a barrier to respite care use, the data collected and subjects studied do not substantiate this view. One project, for example, offered a subsidy with $880 cap; one-third of those eligible for the subsidy did not apply for it. The guide goes on to conclude that "Utilization of temporary, intermittent respite care is not the bottomless pit once envisioned." This is a remarkable conclusion. Where is the study of why family and friend respite caregivers did not apply for meager funds? Where is the finding that they are so worn out that the mere thought of filling in a stack of forms and being interviewed made the stipend not worth the effort? Is policy analysis hibernating?

These are qualitative findings that are not likely to appear in any government-sponsored study. Federal responsibilities have been shifted to state and local governments and to the private sector. "If families are to play any significant role in caring...there will be a growing need for respite services" (Medicare Handbook 1990). Where is the support for the "unpaid caregiver"?*

U.S. Supreme Court Justice Felix Frankfurter once commented, "The mode by which the inevitable is reached is called effort." Finding respite care in New York City is a difficult task even for the experienced. The average consumer needs the services of Lewis and Clark and Jeffersonian providence.

---

* Title III of the Older Americans Act provides very limited help for patients over the age of 60. Some states have adopted expanded in-home services for the elderly but they usually have extremely low income limits. They are often restricted to 72 hours per year. Further, the patient cannot be a Medicaid participant. The income limitation in most cases is less than $8000 per year plus Social Security benefits.

Choices are limited. Public insurance is parsimonious. Private insurance is fledgling. Costs can be prohibitive, even for the wealthiest.

RESPITE CARE IN NEW YORK CITY

What respite care options are available in New York City? What is the cost of 2 weeks of care? This preliminary survey will look at all levels of care—from highly skilled, through intermediate levels, to personal care.

Skilled Care Costs

We will look at one facility that has a formal respite care program. When the need is for highly skilled care, such as for a person with a gastrostomy or someone in a persistent vegetative state, the cost can be more than $200 per day. That means a 2-week respite will cost $2800. Intermediate levels of care are around $150 per day. Intermediate care includes help in activities of daily living such as toileting, transferring and mobility, or care for those with more advanced cognitive dysfunctions. A respite period with this sort of care would cost about $2100.

The above-mentioned facility sets aside two beds for respite care, but this can be increased to nine beds during vacation periods and holidays. Each person admitted needs a patient review (PRI), an electrocardiogram within 90 days, a chest x-ray within 1 year and a complete blood count. The cost of the admission procedure is $125. The length of stay is usually 28 days or less.

If the decision is to have skilled care at home, the cost would probably be out of range for all but the wealthiest. A licensed practical nurse (LPN) can cost $25 to $35 per hour, depending on care requirements. At an average of $30 per hour, a 2-week respite using the services of an LPN will cost a family $10,080. A registered nurse (RN) can cost $40 per hour and up, again depending on care requirements. At an average hourly rate of $45 per hour, that same 2-week respite with an RN would be $15,120.

Home Care Workers

The bulk of home care is done by family members—presumably performed at lower skill levels. What is the cost for health aides and personal care aides? One prominent home care agency's charges for a live-in aide that is *noncertified* is $11.95 per hour with a 5-hour minimum ($59.75). The daily cost is $135 with a minimum of 4 days a week ($540). The weekly cost for a noncertified live-in home health aide is $945. A 2-week respite would cost

$1890. These costs can vary for several reasons: the agency used, the borough in which the care is given, and the level of education of the aide. A *certified* home health aide costs $12.50 per hour. Certified home health aides charge only by the hour; they do not live in. Their daily fee is $300, therefore the weekly charge at this rate would be $2100. Another source of home care workers is registries. Under this program the worker is hired by the family after being screened by the registry. The registry checks references and provides backup assistance. One fee for this service was 18 percent of the first 6 weeks of salary; others charge on a sliding scale. The cost of the aide might be lower, but the family must also pay additional expenses such as insurance, room and board and carfare.

One not-for-profit (NFP) organization places personal care workers for a nominal registration fee. The organization screens both certified and uncertified home attendants, with attention to the linguistic and cultural needs of the Italian community. Personal care—bathing, cooking, dressing, light housekeeping and toileting—is provided by the aides. Referral fees are based on a sliding scale. A typical fee for a live-in aide is $100. The cost of care is $5 to $6 per hour. Live-ins cost $350 to $400 per week, but this does not include room and board. A 2-week respite of this sort would cost $800 plus room and board.

Another private NFP group's formal respite care sends out a certified social worker to assess the needs of the potential client. Participants must be at least 60 years old with minor medical problems. Aides have certificates from a health maintenance school but are not formally certified. Aides are responsible for personal care only, in other words, no money management, no medications. The cost is $5.40 per hour, plus carfare. Care is provided for a maximum of 3 months. The foundation will change the aide if incompatibility arises.

Many families simply use informal neighborhood networks, hiring personal care aides directly. The quality of these aides is uncertain, experience is variable and legal status is sometimes vague. The cost for a live-in can range from $200 to $300 per week. One unique program is the "buddy system" developed by Gay Men's Health Crisis. This organization will match people with AIDS to caregivers when respite is determined to be needed for a few hours, three to four times a week.

Cognitive Illness Respite Support Systems

Families requiring care for a relative with Alzheimer's disease, senile dementia, or other cognitive difficulties have few alternatives. Overnight respite care is available, for example, at the Ridgewood Bushwick Senior Citizen Center. Applicants must be ambulatory; the facility will not accept bedridden patients. There is a six-bed limit. The maximum length of stay is 3 weeks and 2 weeks in the summertime. The center provides bed and board, an RN or LPN from 9:00 a.m. to 5:00 p.m. Monday through Friday, plus a nurse on call on weekends. Medicaid is not accepted. The cost of an overnight stay is $30. A 2-week respite would cost $360.

The care at the Alzheimer's Day Care Program at Aging in America in the Bronx is geared toward those with Alzheimer's disease. Staffed at all times by an RN, the facility is open 7 days a week from 9:30 a.m. to 7:30 p.m. Medicaid is accepted. With the cost of day care at $130 per week, a 2-week respite would be $260.

Care Management

The New York chapter of the National Association of Private Geriatric Care Managers is another resource. Care management can include hands-on home care, filling out Medicaid applications, submitting claims for insurance reimbursement, managing money, transportation and relocation. In addition, some care managers will select, process and monitor home health aides. Costs vary according to tasks. A typical charge is $500 per month; some will have minimum retainer fees. These charges would be in addition to the cost of the aide.

Cost of Care at a Glance

These are the approximate costs for 2 weeks of full-time respite:

Medical Care in a Facility

Type of Care	2 Weeks	Per Annum
Skilled level	$2800	$72,000
Less skilled level	$2100	$54,600

Medical Care at Home

Type of Care	2 Weeks	Per Annum
RN	$15,120	$393,120
LPN	$11,760	$305,760
Certified home health aides	$2000	$52,000
Personal care attendant	$800	$20,800
Care management (monthly)	$500	

Care of Persons with Cognitive Difficulties in a Facility

Type of Care	2 Weeks	Per Annum
Skilled/bedridden	$2800	$72,800
Ambulatory	$360	
Day care	$260	

The second column of numbers, the annual cost, can represent the value of the unpaid caregiver in New York City. At the lowest levels, a family who gives 24-hour care to a loved one in New York City is providing the economic equivalent of $20,800 per year. Is it not in the interest of the public and private sectors to guarantee that this cost not be thrown on the taxpayers's shoulders? By assuring caregivers respite, they can go on.

Medicare and Medicaid

The Medicare provisions have already been outlined. How are Medicare and Medicaid programs applied in New York City? It is more difficult to receive reimbursement for home care services from Medicare than it is to get it from Medicaid. For similar services the Medicare procedural guidelines are more stringent. With the exception of hospice care, Medicare has no respite provision.

Medicaid payments are made after financial limits are met and applications are processed.* Applications for home care are channeled

---

* The application process alone can average 2 months. Under emergency conditions, such as evidence of abuse, the process can be shortened to 2 weeks. If a person is being discharged from a hospital, acceptance can be reduced to 72 hours.

through the Long-Term Health Care Program in New York State. There is no formal respite care provision under the Home Care Program. There are, however, informal applications of its basic principle. For example, a family provides care to their son who has ALS. Medicaid is paying for a limited benefit. The case worker notices that family support may disintegrate or erode due to fatigue. She decides to permit a short-term, 24-hour live-in helper.

Formal respite care is paid under the Lombardi program. There is a dollar cap for the total benefit for the year. The formula for payment for respite is based on a 50 percent cap of the average cost of nursing homes in the county. That is now $2313 per month for skilled care and $1437 per month for nonskilled care. Adult care is paid at 50 percent and home care at 75 to 100 percent of the average cost. There is no cap for hospice care. Admissions to nursing homes for respite care under the Lombardi program require clinical eligibility and are subject to additional Medicare and Medicaid restrictions.

The benefit time limit is 14 days or 336 hours per calendar year. Requests for respite in excess of this limit must have prior approval. In 1990 there was a total of 102 claims for respite care for a total dollar amount of $56,042. This number may not be an accurate representation of total respite claims since some of the charges may have been billed as personal care (e.g., shopping, bathing, meals).

PRIVATE INSURANCE

Major medical insurance provisions for long-term care vary significantly. Generally one will find limited coverage for home care, a maximum number of days of skilled care (usually requiring prior hospitalization) and no custodial care. There are few plans that offer day care, although most cover hospice care. Respite care provisions are rare.

Private Long-Term Care Insurance

Private long-term care insurance is the innovation in options to pay for respite care. More than 130 companies offer this service and more than 1.65 million policies were sold in the United States as of June 1990. Most of the newer generation policies pay for nursing home care at all levels and for home care with restrictions. Many offer benefits for adult day care and hospice care. Some have respite care provisions.

In evaluating the provisions of long-term care insurance contracts as they apply to respite care, we must first consider the following. What is the level of indemnity or reimbursement? What is the waiting or elimination period before benefits begin? Is respite care specifically included? Unless noted otherwise, the contract will have a 20-day waiting period with a $100-a-day indemnity for nursing home care and a respite care provision.

The second major consideration is the eligibility trigger in the contract. Most newer policies have benefits that are triggered by activities of daily living (ADL) criteria. This is usually disability in two or three out of five or six ADLs, including eating, dressing, transferring, mobility, maintaining continence, toileting and cognitive impairment. Others will require physician certification or a determination of medical necessity.

The third consideration is the qualifying nature of the services used. Will the provider be recognized under law and contract? The use of uncertified care workers, social day care models or congregate living facilities may not be covered. In addition, the licensing requirements for providers of adult day care may vary from state to state.

Respite Care Provisions

Respite care provisions are new. The benefit for respite care is usually for a maximum number of days per year times the daily nursing home or home care benefit to a maximum dollar figure per year. For example, if the policy pays $100 per day indemnity with a respite provision of 14 days, the maximum benefit would be $1400 per year. Some contracts may limit the respite care benefit to the level of care. If, using the same example, a person is receiving home care at 50 percent of the daily indemnity, then the respite payout would be $700 per year or one-half of the maximum payout for home care. If this amount is not enough to cover the cost of home care, the policyholder may wish to use a qualified facility for care, thereby receiving the higher indemnity ($1400).

In our review, the number of days of respite care covered ranged from 14 to 21 days. The total benefit was usually in addition to the current benefit (depending on level of care), but not more than the actual charge.

There are additional requirements. There is an assumption that a claim has been filed and that the claimant is eligible to receive care at home or in an adult care facility, or home hospice care. If a nursing home is to be used for respite, then the requirements of eligibility under the contract and the admission criteria of the nursing home must be met. There is also an assumption that the family is providing unpaid caregiving services. Would the benefit be paid to nonfamily caregivers?

One of the more interesting issues is the nature of the waiting period for most policies. There is substantial variance. Will the benefit trigger after the waiting period, or after *no* waiting period? If there is no waiting period for respite care will this benefit be used as a post-acute coverage (e.g., for post-hospitalization short-term care)? With a shorter waiting period will the benefit be misutilized? Respite care provisions in long-term care insurance contracts are an untested boon to unpaid caregivers.

CONCLUSION

If caring for the chronically ill is an emotional abyss, it is a financial nightmare. Our society's emphasis on curing over caring provides a fragile and fragmented resource network to these individuals and their caregivers. Enhanced private and public programs for respite care will prolong the valuable economic contributions made by family and friends. Innovation, such as respite care provisions in long-term care insurance, is crucial for future needs. Caregivers need to have resources to return, in the words of Dorothy L. Sayers, "To that still center where the spinning world \ Sleeps on its axis, to the heart of rest."

REFERENCES

Callahan, D. *What Kind of Life?* New York: 1990.
Eisenberg, L. The search for care. *Daedalus* 106:3-38, 1977.
Malcolm, A.H. *This Far and No More.* New York: 1987.
Medicare Handbook. Washington, DC: U.S. Department of Health and Human Services, 1990.
National Institutes of Health. *Amyotrophic Lateral Sclerosis: Hope Through Research.* Publication No. 84-16. Rockville, MD: NIH, 1984.

12

Dementia Day Care: Respite or Therapy?

Elizabeth Ryan, RN, Ronald S. Black, MD, Karen Nolan, PhD, Margaret Trahar, MS, RN and John Blass, MD

Day care programs for patients with dementia have been recognized as one way of providing care and managing such patients and at the same time maintaining them in the community. Research in respite care has attempted to determine if such care can prevent nursing home placement and how the use of respite care affects caregivers in terms of stress. The results of these studies are conflicting. For example, Chodosh and co-workers (1986) described a medical day program for patients with dementia in which approximately 26 percent of their initial sample eventually sought nursing home placement. This rate was attributed to the effectiveness of the program. But in a much larger sample, Lawton and associates (1989) found that 317 caregivers who were offered some type of respite care (overnight nursing home placement, home care or day care) were able to keep the patient with dementia home only 3 weeks longer than the control group that was not offered such services. In other words, use of respite services did not prevent nursing home placement, but only postponed it for a very short time. The findings of the aforementioned studies have yielded a confused picture of the effects of participation in a day care program in terms of nursing home placement.

Studies that examine caregiver burden have yielded similarly mixed results. Although it has been clearly documented that caregivers do experience burden (Zarit et al. 1980; Rabins et al. 1982), it is less certain whether day care provides temporary relief as Strang and Neufeld found, or if it can diminish caregiver stress as Looney reports. Mohide and co-workers found regular in-home respite did not affect caregiver depression or anxiety but did result in a perceived improvement of quality of life and management of the patient. Respite use (overnight nursing home, placement, home assistance, or day care) did not alleviate caregiver burden or improve caregiver well-being (Lawton, Brody and Saperstein 1989). Caregivers of dementia patients who were enrolled in a day program did not experience significantly less stress (Graham 1989).

Despite the conflicting data regarding the effect of day care use, some caregivers continue to utilize such programs. Since it is unclear why caregivers use such programs, we decided to do a pilot study that investigated their reasons for using day care by means of a questionnaire.

METHOD

Sample

The initial sample included 31 caregivers of patients enrolled in the Senior Day Care Program (medical model) at Burke Rehabilitation Center in White Plains, New York. The response rate was 89 percent. All patients were diagnosed with a dementing illness. To ascertain the generalizability of responses to this questionnaire, caregivers of attendees of the Central Westchester Senior Day Center (psychosocial model) were also surveyed. Data were obtained from 17 of these caregivers and the response rate was 55 percent. The only selection factor was caring for a family member who attended a dementia day care program.

Of the Burke group 45 percent of the respondents were spouses, another 45 percent were daughters and the others were sisters. The respondents were mostly women (87 percent). In the Central Westchester sample half of the respondents were men and half were women; 65 percent were spouses. More than half of the patients in each program were women. The patients in each of the programs had a variety of dementing illnesses. Alzheimer's disease was the most common diagnosis in each group. There were nearly twice as many patients with multi-infarct dementia in the Burke population as in the Central Westchester one. Patients diagnosed as having some other form of dementia were nearly equal for the two groups.

Instrument

Caregivers of Burke and Central Westchester patients were asked to respond to a questionnaire designed to measure how useful day care was to them. The questionnaire mailed to the caregivers by the Senior Day

Care Center at Burke Rehabilitation Center consisted of ten open-ended questions and included items such as reasons for attendance, the importance of the program to the family schedule, how the patient spent time when not attending program and the caregiver's use of supportive services. Logistical inquiries about method of referral and family method of payment were also made. And finally caregivers were asked to predict both their response to a hypothetical fee increase on attendance. Which services families would use in place of the program were it not available. The Central Westchester sample was mailed a revised questionnaire that in addition to the ten questions from the original questionnaire included demographic information, patient diagnosis and the date the patient began attending the program. Caregivers were also asked how they felt the program affected patient behavior or illness.

RESULTS

Families' reasons for using day care, while varied, showed some interesting similarities. The most frequently reported reason was to give the patient a chance to socialize and engage in activities. As Table 1 indicates, respite, caregiver employment and the need for the patient to be supervised were also mentioned. Some other reasons for attending the program were the physician's recommendation, patient enjoyment of the program, slowing of disease progression and improvement of the patient's quality of life.

In addition to the reason for attendance, Central Westchester caregivers were also asked how they felt the program affected patient behavior or illness (Table 2). Thirty-five percent of the caregivers reported it helped the patient to continue to socialize and be active, while 25 percent said it made the patient happy. Some 20 percent of families were not sure and 10 percent saw little change. Five percent of the caregivers reported it slowed the patient's deterioration and another 5 percent said it made the patient more alert and manageable. By combining the 25 percent of caregivers who reported that participation made the patient happy with the 5 percent who said the patient was more alert and manageable and the 5 percent who reported that participation slowed the patient's deterioration, a total of 35 percent of the caregivers reported a beneficial effect on patient behavior.

When caregivers were asked what alternate arrangements could be made if the present day care program was no longer available, each sample differed in the frequency of their responses, as shown in Table 3. Most caregivers in the Burke group were unsure what service (if any) they would use in place of the present program, whereas almost half of the

Central Westchester caregivers would choose an in-home companion as a substitute for day care.

More than half of the families in each sample were private payers. One third of the Burke patients received Medicaid assistance and two families from Central Westchester received assistance from an Alzheimer's Association grant. More than one third of the families from both Burke and Central Westchester were willing to pay more for day care. However, the Central Westchester respondents wanted to see the program fully Medicaid-approved. The Burke caregivers suggested that patients be allowed to attend more days (the maximum was 4) when asked how the program could be improved.

DISCUSSION

These findings indicate there is more than one determinant to day care placement. Twice as many caregivers in each sample cited the opportunity for socialization and activities rather than caregiver respite as the reason for patient participation. The motive of many caregivers seems to have an altruistic component. The families saw day care as a therapeutic agent that helped patients continue to socialize, a function they could no longer initiate independently. They saw the replacement of this function through day care as reason enough to attend. While the Rabins and Chodosh teams found that caregivers preferred to care for the patient at home, we found day care to have a dual benefit because it structures a patient's day and this helps the caregiver to maintain the patient at home. We believe the therapeutic goal of day care may be to maintain the patient's person-hood by providing a structured environment in which to socialize.

Although caregivers may see participation in day care as therapeutic, few (10 percent) reported any improvement in patient behavior. Studies of day care confirm that it cannot halt disease progression (Chodosh et al. 1986; Panella et al. 1984) and research that supports improved behavior is based on subjective reporting (Chodosh et al. 1986; Sands and Suzuki 1983). In Sands and Suzuki's work, estimates of patient improvements were based on caregiver reports which the authors corroborated and in the work of Chodosh and co-workers, improvements were reported by the day care staff.

Since this study is based on subjective reports of the caregiver, it may be possible that the caregiver is the recipient of the therapeutic value of day care participation. Caregivers may choose to believe that day program activities are beneficial in order to justify using the programs without feeling selfish. For some caregivers, it may be difficult to admit to the need for respite. Future research should focus on whether the caregivers who

Table 1.

Reasons for Attendance

	Burke	Central Westchester
Socialization/Activities	40%	55%
Respite	20%	30%
Caregiver works	10%	11%
Need supervision	18%	4%
Other	12%	

Table 2.

Alternate Arrangements

	Burke	Central Westchester
Not sure	27%	26%
Home health aide	23%	47%
None	13%	11%
Another day program	20%	11%
Nursing home	17%	5%

Table 3.

How Participation Affected Behavior

Helped patient to socialize	35%
Made patient happy	25%
Not sure	20%
Little change	10%
Made patient more alert	5%
Slowed patient's decline	5%

perceive benefit are those whose family members do benefit cognitively, behaviorally or in terms of mood.

Targeting respite to the population for whom it is intended would be worthwhile, considering the results of this study. Although this sample is biased toward a middle-class, suburban population in which 50 percent are private payers, socialization and activities are what these caregivers want from day care. While the results presented here may not be duplicated with a different sample, this study clearly shows the value of service delivery that is focused on what the caregiver desires for the patient. Follow-up studies on targeting day care services should focus on determining which aspects of a program are important and whether patients benefit differently depending on how a program is structured. It remains unclear whether day care truly decreases caregiver burden or prevents nursing home placement. It may, however, benefit the caregivers simply by enhancing their perception of the patient's quality of life.

REFERENCES

Chodosh, H.L., B. Zeffert and E.S. Muro. Treatment of dementia in a medical day program. *J. Am. Geriatrics Soc.* 34(12):881-886, 1988.

Graham, R.W. Adult day care: how families of the dementia patient respond. *J. Gerontol. Nursing* 15(3):27-31, 1988.

Lawton, M.P., E.M. Brody and A.R. Saperstein. A controlled study of respite service for caregivers of Alzheimer's patients. *Gerontologist* 29(1):8-16, 1989.

Looney, K.M. The respite care alternative. *J. Gerontol. Nursing* 13(5):18-21, 1989.

Mohide, E.A., D.M. Pringle, D.L. Streiner, J.R. Gilbert, G. Muir and M. Tew. A randomized trial of family caregiver support in the home management of dementia. *J. Am. Geriatrics Soc.* 38(4):446-453, 1990.

Panella, J.J., B.A. Lilliston, D. Brush and F.H. McDowell. Day care for dementia patients: analysis of a four-year program. *J. Am. Geriatrics Soc.* 32(12):883-886, 1984.

Rabins, P.V., N.L. Mace, and M.J. Lucas. The impact of dementia on the family. *JAMA* 248(3):333-335, 1982.

Sands, D. and T. Suzuki. Adult day care for Alzheimer's patients and their families. *Gerontologist* 23(1):21-23, 1983.

Strang, V. and A. Neufeld. Adult day care programs: a source for respite. *J. Gerontol. Nursing* 16(11):16-19, 1989.

Zarit, S.H., K.E. Reeves and J. Bach-Peterson. Relatives of impaired elderly: correlates of feelings of burden. *Gerontologist* 20:649-655, 1980.

Concepts of Respite Care

13

Respite as Treatment

Shura Saul, EdD, BCD, CSW

We generally think of respite as a time of "temporary relief or rest from pain, work or duty...a putting off of something fixed, especially of something disagreeable" (Webster 1988). We may all agree on the value of a "time hiatus" in which pressuring emotions are mitigated, difficult mental activities are put on hold and energies are replenished. On a personal level, most of us have had a range of opportunities with a variety of respite experiences—whether in the form of caregiving or from other arduous activities. We all appreciate the value of the chance to get away from our daily responsibilities, especially a duty such as caregiving which is charged with emotion.

The best professional efforts have recognized that spending respite time alone is not enough. How we use time and what we do during these times matter greatly. Therefore, during times of respite, consultation may often be useful for the family as is providing information on various forms of treatment available to the patient. This chapter addresses an additional component that enhances the traditional value of the respite concept— respite as a part of treatment in community psychiatry care.

The programs with which I am most familiar are conducted in Scotland, where I had the good fortune to work for several periods over 10 years. In particular, I will describe the Community Psychiatry Program of Dingleton Hospital in Melrose, where Dr. Maxwell Jones developed his model of the therapeutic community. His initial work within this mental hospital has been extended into the four shires of the hospital's catchment area. Both prevention and treatment are provided to residents of these shires through a range of community psychiatry programs.

This program emphasizes early intervention and continuity of care, both of which grow out of a unique working relationship between the attending physician in the community and the outreach psychiatric team of the mental hospital. In recognition of his primary role, the family physician chairs the community team which meets periodically to review individual patient cases, assess new needs and adjust treatment plans accordingly. With such teamwork between family physician and hospital psychiatric staff (psychiatrist, psychiatric nurse and psychiatric social worker, all of whom participate actively in the community program, leaving the hospital to meet in the community, making home visits as needed), respite becomes an additional treatment modality, one that may be recommended for the patient and the family. In this program, the family is seen as primary caregiver and treatment agent and is involved as much as possible in the planning of care. Wherever appropriate, the patient is similarly involved.

The approach to treatment is multidisciplinary: the treatment plan is related to physical, psychological, social and emotional needs. Treatment modalities may include: medical and pharmaceutical interventions; speech, hearing, or physical and occupational therapies; psychiatric treatment or psychosocial programs; group or individual methods. The plan may include any or all of these, as well as any other modalities that may be indicated to treat dysfunction or enhance the quality of the patient's and the family's life.

The hospital team regards all relevant community agents as possible collaborators in psychosocial treatment. When appropriate, members of the community—clergy, storekeepers, police personnel, postmen, even the local bartender—may be drawn into the treatment and support plan.

When we first came to Dingleton Hospital and began to study case material of patients with whom we would be working, we found background material reflecting many years of contact with patients and families prior to hospital admission, sometimes as far back as 10 to 15 years.

This important information had two sources: treatment at home by the outreach psychiatric team working in concert with the family physician and treatment in the hospital during the weeks of respite spent years before admission. Thus the time that the patient spent in the hospital, time that also provides respite for the family, becomes a time of treatment and continuity in the ongoing care plan for the chronically ill patient. During this time, the patient's condition is re-evaluated, new treatment or medications prescribed and follow-up in the community planned for when the patient goes home.

EXAMPLES

Case 1

Mrs. A.'s family was anticipating a 2-week vacation and requested respite care for their mother while they were away. Incidentally, this is seen as both the family's right and the patient's right, and it is viewed as an integral dimension of treatment. Mrs. A. had been a patient in the community psychiatry program and this referral for respite came from her family physician. The need had been anticipated somewhat earlier in a community-based team meeting. A pre-respite home visit by the hospital team was attended by Mrs. A. and her family. The family described the most recent changes in their mother's condition and her current behavior at home. She had, for example, recently become incontinent. They noted also that she was no longer able to make her wishes clear. She had begun to wander and would get lost when alone out of doors. She also wandered about the house during the night. These were new developments, and the family was finding it very difficult to cope. Mrs. A. was becoming angry at the restrictions the family had begun to set.

The psychiatrist and social worker (in this case, a psychiatric nurse was involved) agreed to admit Mrs. A. They arranged the transportation and suggested that the family accompany Mrs. A. to the hospital. Mrs. A. was admitted for 2 weeks during which time she was evaluated, appropriate examinations and tests were administered, and a new treatment plan developed. When the family returned, refreshed from their holiday, they were advised of these developments, and suggestions were made for their continued role as caregivers within the new plan. Follow-up visits were made by the psychiatric nurse on the team, who communicated regularly with the family physician.

Case 2

Mr. C. was living alone, a few doors down the street from his daughter who looked after him. At a community team meeting, the attending physician reported that Mr. C. had been awakening during the night, walking out of the house and going from nearby farm to farm opening the gates and releasing the farm animals who had to be rounded up each morning. Clearly, the whole town needed some respite from Mr. C.

Mr. C. was admitted for a respite period (coinciding with his daughter's holiday), evaluated, and a treatment plan developed. When his daughter returned, the team, including the family physician, met with her and with Mr. C. and developed a home care plan. Among other recommendations, Mr. C. was referred for attendance at a day treatment program conducted by the hospital in his community. A follow-up home visit by the team confirmed that the plans were in place and Mr. C. was doing well.

These examples show clearly the enhanced value of respite when (1) all treatment agents and caring persons work together on behalf of the patient; (2) communication is professionally focused on needs and treatment; (3) patient condition is monitored on an ongoing basis through appropriate sharing among family, family physician and hospital team; (4) the patient is involved as much as possible and (5) continuity of care and close articulation of treatment are fitted appropriately into the life of the patient and the family.

The model described here is applicable to the care of a dependent family member of any age—and certainly for elderly parents who are being cared for at home. While the specifics of this model may not be replicable in all its detail within the long-term care system in the United States, the vision of respite as a component of treatment and continuity can conceivably be implemented in other ways. A variety of adaptations of this approach is possible when the basic philosophy of care, concern and teamwork prevails.

14

Concepts of Respite Care: A Gerontologist's Perspective

John A. Toner, EdD

The focus of this chapter is concepts of respite that have evolved from personal and professional experiences. Although I have given some attention to technical aspects of respite—organizational structures, funding mechanisms and successful models of respite—these are covered in greater depth in other chapters of this book.

Knowledge of respite, for most gerontologists, is shaped almost entirely by what is reported in the professional and scientific literature. Until recently (especially during my formative years as a gerontologist in the early 1970s), very little was published about respite, particularly in the scientific literature. From the early 1980s to the present, my knowledge of respite has been shaped by personal experience, both as a respite care provider and as a primary caregiver needing respite.

My experience as a respite care provider began in 1981 after I returned to New York from a 6-month voyage around the world. Upon arriving home, I learned that while I was away my father had suffered a heart attack, developed life-threatening complications and had been hospitalized for nearly 2 months, part of which time he in a comatose state and on a respirator. At the beginning of his hospitalization he insisted that no one contact me about his illness under any circumstance. Like me, my father had just returned home from a trip, but his voyage had left him severely impaired, frail and unable to walk. The year that followed was filled with some physical gains for my father, but for the most part he experienced heavy losses of physical abilities. Through it all, my disabled arthritic mother insisted on providing for my father's personal care, in spite of the fact that nurses and health aides were being paid to deliver such care. The only people that my mother—and, by the way, my father, also—would allow to provide my father with personal care were her sons. So that is how I came to learn about providing respite care services. I would give my mother respite from caring for my father during the weekends and I had respite during the remainder of the week.

My experience as primary caregiver needing respite began 3 years after the onset of my father's debilitating illness. My father had passed away and my 76-year-old unmarried aunt and 90-year-old grandmother came to live with my mother, who had been living alone since my father's death. Although my mother's new living arrangement was not working well, no one could have dreamed what was in store for our family. One early morning in April, my mother's home was completely destroyed by an explosion and subsequent fire. Fortunately, no one was home at the time. Because of my close relationship with my aunt and grandmother and because I lived in a large three-bedroom apartment on the Upper West Side of New York City, I suggested that they come and stay with me for a couple of weeks. Little did I know that 2 weeks would turn into nearly 3 months and that life with Nana and Aunt Catherine would read like the script from Auntie Mame. Regardless, I became a primary caregiver with an extreme need for respite. The way in which my respite manifested itself was in the form of business trips. It seemed like I was constantly traveling. Upon my return home after a business trip I was inevitably greeted at the door by my grandmother, who would sheepishly inform me of my aunt's latest shenanigans. "Don't say anything to Aunt Catherine," she would say to me as she unlocked and opened the apartment door, "but we had a little fire while you were gone. No one was hurt and those firemen, well they're such fine boys." On another occasion I returned home from a weekend of reviewing grant proposals in Washington, D.C. to learn that "Auntie" had managed to lock one of the apartment doors for which there was no key. It was jammed in the locked position and required the services of a very skilled locksmith to open it. Auntie's only comment was, "a fine boy that locksmith." My girlfriend (later to become my wife) had her share of experiences as well. It wasn't easy at first explaining to my Irish Catholic grandmother that my girlfriend didn't go home when the lights were turned out at night.

Eventually, the day came for my grandmother and aunt to return to New Jersey. I continued to be the primary caregiver, but provided support services at a distance; regularly traveling to New Jersey to shop for Auntie and Nana, take them to appointments or visits with friends. Over the next few years these trips became more frequent and more crisis-oriented. The rate of falls, fractures and hospitalizations increased. Fortunately, we had secondary caregivers in the form of my mother and brothers to provide respite services for my wife and myself. Eventually, we decided to move out of our apartment in New York to the town where my grandmother and aunt lived. Within a month of our move, my aunt was diagnosed with metastatic lung cancer. Within the year she was dead. Then, the following year my grandmother died at the age of 97.

For many in the fields of geriatrics and gerontology, the concepts of respite have evolved in very much the same manner as they did for me, both professionally and personally, as a member of the so-called sandwich generation. Before elaborating on this theme and describing how the 9-year-long respite experience described above relates to the evolution of respite concepts, it is first necessary to define "respite care" and briefly trace the recent history of formal respite services. From this background information, a theoretical framework will be described. This theoretical framework is one of the two concepts on which this chapter focuses, and it represents my personal and professional perspective. The roots of this perspective are found in the sociological literature, particularly in Eugene Litwak's theory of formal organizations and primary group structures (Litwak 1985).

DEFINITION OF TERMS

Most definitions of respite care share the notion that it is temporary or intermittent substitute care which provides relief to the primary caregiver, who typically performs most of the care for the older person with others who take distinctly secondary roles (Gwyther 1986). Hasselkus and Brown (1983) expand this definition and indicate that respite care is *planned* intermittent, short-term care designed to provide periodic relief to the family and caregivers "from the 24-hour continuous care of the frail family member." This can mean care that is given in the home setting (for example, a volunteer may come for short periods during the day to relieve the caregivers) or at a community day care center. Respite care can also include a program of short-term hospitalization to provide longer periods of rest for the patient and for his family. Such programs of respite are really aimed at keeping the ill, disabled or frail elderly person in the community and out of nursing homes for longer periods of time. It is hoped that by accomplishing this goal, the life of aged people will be enhanced (Hasselkus and Brown 1983).

The underlying assumption is that the primary caregiver experiences significant stress due to the unremitting provision of care and that respite care provides temporary relief that reduces the stress on the primary caregiver. This form of respite care is most often provided by informal caregivers, primarily members of the primary group (e.g., family, friends and sometimes neighbors), and is referred to as *informal respite care*. Another form of respite care which receives the majority of attention in the scientific literature is *formal respite care*. Formal care refers to the provision of such care by those who are not a part of the primary group just mentioned; instead it is provided formally by a facility (in-home aides, hospitals, hospices, adult day care programs, etc).

BRIEF HISTORY OF RESPITE

Although there are certainly examples of respite or respite-like services provided to families of the chronically ill elderly throughout much of this century, indeed throughout most of history, the legitimization of respite as a specific type of formal services for the elderly did not occur until the mid to late 1970s when a number of articles on the topic of respite were published in the scientific literature.

The increased concern regarding the role of the family in caring for the chronically ill elderly led to the early studies of family caregiving characteristics (Shanas 1979). This, in turn, led to the early studies of caregiver burden (Lebowitz 1978) and work on old age and family functioning (Fengler and Goodrich 1979), and ultimately to studies of how formal services might reduce caregiver stress by providing relief from caregiving responsibilities (Rathbone-McCuan 1976; Horowitz 1978). The acknowledgment of the critical role that families play in the care of their older family members and the need that family members have for formal services to supplement the care they deliver eventually led to the development of formal respite services.

It just so happened that at about the same time (late 1970s and early 1980s), adult day care programs began to emerge as a long-term care option. Although not originally conceived of as a respite service, adult day care has evolved as a legitimate form of respite.

EVOLVING CONCEPTS OF RESPITE CARE

Formal Respite Services

Even though the primary focus of this chapter is informal respite services, a brief overview of formal respite services will be useful. There are three major forms of formal respite services.

    1. *In-home sitter/companions* are paid workers or volunteers who provide

respite services for periods of time ranging from hours to days. The respite worker usually has no formal training and may be hired through the same sort of informal network that is used to find babysitters for children. Supervision and companionship are provided, a simple meal may be prepared and occasionally bathing may be provided.

2. *Adult day care* is community-based respite that provides various types of services depending on the population being served. Among other services, adult day care programs provide patients with the opportunity for socialization with peers and activities in a structured setting. These programs are regulated by state and local agencies and must meet certain minimum staff and facility requirements.

3 *Overnight or short-term residential respite* is provided in a variety of institutional facilities, including skilled nursing homes, intermediate care facilities, adult residences, Veterans Hospitals and senior housing. One of the potential advantages of residential respite is the array of social and personal services available in most residential settings.

Informal Networks as a Source of Respite

In spite of the fact that caregiver studies routinely report high levels of caregiver stress related to the burden of providing care and in spite of the fact that surveys (Seagall and Wykle 1988-89) indicate that caregivers long for respite services, studies indicate that respite services are often underutilized. Although the demand appears great, the utilization of formal respite services provides evidence to the contrary. In fact, Lawton and Brody report that in their controlled study of respite services for caregivers of Alzheimer's patients, only half of their subjects actually used the respite services that were offered even when these services were offered at no cost, and transportation was included (Lawton, Brody and Saperstein 1989).

If the need for respite services is well documented, why are they being underutilized? The most obvious answer to this question is that informal networks are meeting the needs of the chronically ill and the impaired elderly and therefore the demand for formal respite services is low.

In order to understand why people choose informal care, it would be helpful to understand and apply Eugene Litwak's model of formal organizations and primary group structures. In the model, Litwak compares and contrasts formal organizations (we can substitute formal respite services) and primary group structures (for our purposes, respite services provided by the informal network) in terms of recruitment, commitment and tasks.

Informal Group Structures

	Formal	*Informal*
Recruitment	Technical knowledge	Birth/marriage/ friendshi[p
Commitment	Limited; based most often on fee for service	Long-term/life; based on internalized level of commitment; duty and love
Tasks	Technical skills	Skills developed through socialization; companionship; assistance with basic and instrumental activities

It is clear that informal networks, particularly primary groups, provide the bulk of respite services to primary caregivers of the elderly and chronically ill (Stone 1987). It is also clear that this limits the demand for formal respite programs. The primary group or informal network accomplishes this in three ways:

1. Diffusion of the primary caregiver's stress, which in turn enables that person to continue caregiving until another crisis arises.
2. Provision of emotional support and supplementary assistance with basic and instrumental activities of daily living, which reduces the need for formal respite services.
3. Serving as the primary caregiver's only referral source to the outside world.

CONCLUSIONS

In order to properly plan programs of respite care it is important to know who these programs should be aimed at helping. Thus, it is necessary to look at who is giving long-term care to dependent elderly in the community. Due to the persistent sex-role differences and the longer female life expectancy, women have been found to be much more likely than men to assume the task of providing care to the elderly person. The exception to this is the case of elderly married couples, in which the wife is disabled or ill. In this case, the husband will most often assume traditional "female" caregiving tasks (Shanas 1979).

Today, with the high cost of living and the high number of single parent homes, there are increasing numbers of women joining the workforce who would otherwise be at home caring for their elderly parents or other relatives. This has had a dramatic effect on the ability of families to care for an elderly relative. This has implications not only in regard to the increased stress placed on the family unit, but also on the competing demands placed on working women to provide the care needed care by their aged relatives and concurrently to perform adequately in their full-time job. The problem is further complicated by the fact that such female caregivers bear the responsibility of maintaining their own households, which itself is usually a full-time effort. Newman (1976) found that nearly two-fifths of the children caring for their aged parents were spending the equivalent of a full day's work per week performing caregiving tasks.

Caring for an elderly relative in the home is often provided at great cost to a family's psychological, physical and financial resources. Zarit and co-workers (1980) report that the extent of the burden felt and expressed by caregivers was not related to the behavior problems of the elderly person, but rather to the degree to which social supports to provide respite were available.

The following conclusions regarding the need, underutilization and future of respite care draw heavily on my personal and professional perspectives:

1. Cultural and ethnic values, attitudes and norms play a crucial role in caretakers' seeking formal services and utilizing them appropriately. In the example of my father's case, given at the beginning of this chapter, the primary caregiver, my mother, would not allow health care workers to provide the very physically demanding personal care he needed, even though these health care workers were being paid and were very willing to provide this care.

2. The involvement of secondary caregivers increases the likelihood of formal service utilization. In each of the examples cited at the beginning of this chapter, when other family members became involved with care, the primary caregiver was more responsive to seeking more formal respite services.

3. My professional perspective regarding caregiving and respite care has changed as a result of my personal experience with caregiving and the long-term care system. What I once considered a clear-cut model of service utilization (i.e., increased impairment leads to

increased caregiver burden and stress, which further leads to the use of formal respite services, which ultimately leads to institution-alization) is not clear-cut at all. The decision to use formal respite services is very complicated and idiosyncratic and warrants more scientific investigation.

4. Primary caregiver distress, which would most often lead to utiliza-tion of formal respite services, is extremely variable even among the caregivers of very impaired elderly. For instance, the level of distress that my mother experienced providing care to her dying sister was much greater than that which she experienced providing care for my father, even though the physical demands of caring for my father were greater.

5. The manner in which we perceive ourselves as caregivers has much to do with the level of our distress. This can be seen in each of the examples discussed at the beginning of this chapter. In my father's case, my absence during the entire time of his acute illness intensi-fied my sense of obligation during the subsequent chronic phase of his illness—when I was accessible. In my aunt's and grandmother's cases, long-standing relationships helped me to differentiate my feelings about caregiver tasks and about caring for a loved one.

6. The experiences of providing respite care as a secondary caregiver and needing respite as a primary caregiver have helped me, as a gerontologist, to recognize how little we know about meeting the respite needs of caregivers.

REFERENCES

Fengler, A. and N. Goodrich. Wives of elderly disabled men: the hidden patients. *Gerontologist* 19:175-183, 1979.

Gwyther, L. Introduction: what is respite care? *Pride Inst. J. Long-Term Home Health Care* 5:4-6, 1986.

Hasselkus, B. and M. Brown. Respite care for community elderly. *Am. J. Occup. Ther.* 37:83-88, 1983.

Horowitz, A. Families who care: a study of natural support systems of the elderly. Paper presented at the Annual Scientific Meeting of the Gerontological Society, November 1978.

Lawton, P., E. Brody and A. Saperstein. A controlled study of respite service for caregivers of Alzheimer's patients. *Gerontologist* 29:8-16, 1989.

Lebowitz, B. Old age and family functioning. *J. Gerontol. Social Work* 1:111-118, Winter, 1978.

Litwak, E. *Helping the Elderly: The Complementary Role of Informal Networks and Formal Systems.* New York: Guilford Press, 1985.

Newman, S. *Housing Adjustments of Older People: A Report from the Second* Phase. Ann Arbor, MI: Institute for Social Research, 1976.

Rathbone-McCuan, E. Geriatric day care: a family perspective. *Gerontologist* 16:517-521, 1976.

Segall, M. and M. Wykle. The black families' experience with dementia. *J. App. Soc. Sci.* 13:170-191, 1988-89.

Shanas, E. The family as a social support system in old age. *Gerontologist* 19:169-174, 1979.

Stone, R. National profile of caregivers. *Gerontologist* 27:616-631, 1987.

Zarit, S., K. Reeves and J. Bach-Peterson. Relatives of the impaired elderly: correlates of feelings of burden. *Gerontologist* 20:649-654. 1980.

15

Respite for the Alzheimer's Patient and Family: A Psychosocial Treatment Program

Sidney R. Saul, EdD, BCD, CSW

The traditional frame of reference for the concept of respite refers to the needs of the family and the caregivers of the very ill patient. However, the task of caring for an Alzheimer's patient at home suggests that this concept requires a more comprehensive approach, one that is extended to include the needs of the patient as well. The program described below was developed to provide much needed respite for the patient, as well as for the family and other caring persons.

Inasmuch as more than half of the victims of Alzheimer's disease live in the community and are being cared for at home by their families, it is important to review some aspects of the home and family situation and relationships that generally develop when a family member has this particular disease. Known as the "Silent Epidemic," this disease progresses stealthily and quietly and may develop over a period of 10 to more than 15 years. Clearly, this is a long-term, chronic illness for which there is still no known medical treatment. Thus it creates an increasing and progressive problem for the family as well as for the patient.

Let us consider how the onset of Alzheimer's disease in one member of a family affects the entire family system—especially when the family is caring and involved. Briefly stated, it has the emotional impact of tearing the family apart. More specifically, watching a loved one who has always been a capable, competent, intelligent and a socially involved person gradually deteriorate may well induce, within the caregivers, a range of emotional responses such as anger, tension, guilt, anxiety, frustration and social isolation.

Also, the cruel changes in the patient's personality and cognitive abilities that this illness causes have a cruel effect upon the feelings of caregivers. The caring spouse becomes a slave to a stranger, since the victim loses all resemblance to his former self—the husband of 50 years who regards his wife as a total stranger, or the wife who tells her husband of 40 years that there is a strange man who comes to her bedroom every night.

Other personality changes develop, along with erratic, difficult and sometimes even abusive and assaultive behavior. The family may become confused and baffled and often either does not know how to cope with the problems, or they become totally unable to do so. It is rare for the family of an Alzheimer's patient not to suffer from both the emotional and physical strains of caregiving.

Another common characteristic of the behavior of Alzheimer's patients is restlessness and a tendency to wander. This is especially dangerous as the patient, at this stage of this progressive disease, may well have forgotten his name, address and other identifying data. Alzheimer's patients have been known to disappear from home for long periods of time before being found. Fearful of this possibility, families tend to lock doors and windows as it is practically impossible to watch the home-bound patient every minute. Thus, both the caring person and the patient become prisoners in their own home.

This tension and strain upon the family members may often result in inappropriate expectations of the patient. These are extended both verbally and nonverbally. On the one hand, questions arise such as, "Why can't he control his bladder?" "She always knew her phone number, why not now?" and "She should be able to pick up her own clothes and dress herself."

On the other hand, the caring family may be infantilizing the patient; for example, the caregiver may feed the person, rather than encourage self-feeding. Because of the patient's confusion, the caregiver may perform a variety of activities of daily living that the patient might well be able to perform himself. These double messages can exacerbate the existing confusion felt by patients. The ill person may have his own expectations of the family or caregivers—expectations that may well be as inappropriate as are those that the family has for him.

The combination of the patient's confused communication, inappropriate expectations, altered relationships and diminished functioning usually results in tremendous frustration for both patient and family. It may also account for the abusive and even violent behavior exhibited by some Alzheimer's patients in the advanced stages of the illness.

All too common are the breakup of marriages of long standing, or close-knit families falling apart as children and grandchildren become angry with each other. The question, "How come I get stuck with the old lady?" is heard all too often. And in the midst of all this turmoil is the patient. In their contact with Alzheimer's patients, most professionals, as well as caregivers, have learned that no matter how disoriented and confused the patient may be, their emotional feelings remain quite perceptive. The patient feels another's anger, approval and acceptance, pressure or support, rejection and love. It is from this "battlefield of emotions" that the patient needs respite, as does the family.

The program described here is a multifaceted treatment/diagnostic/teaching program that operates as a day hospital service, 5 days a week, for 5 hours a day (which includes travel time). We recognize that we cannot treat the disease, but we can treat the patient. We can treat the patient's depression, the overwhelming anxiety and the loss of impulse and behavior controls. We can treat the patient's loss of sense-of-self and sense-of-competence. We may not be able to cure, but we can treat, ease and modify affect and behavior. This group program provides several important benefits for the patient:

1. It fosters peer experiences and emotional support through group interaction and supportive, compassionate group leadership.
2. It stimulates, encourages and supports the functioning of all available, remaining intellectual and social capacities. It makes maximum use of available memory and motivates cognitive functioning and socialization.
3. It evokes positive emotions and affect within the group situation.
4. It affirms and confirms a sense of individual identity which actively combats the tendency to lose sense-of-self.
5. It offers an ego-supportive experience.
6. It gives the patient unqualified acceptance, tenderness and kind treatment by a staff carefully trained to do so.
7. By eliminating frustrating expectations and replacing them with positive, supportive social and group control, it elicits the best possible level of social behavior and the highest possible cognitive response of each individual patient. (Consequently there has rarely been an incident of abusive or assaultive behavior in the group program.)

This program may be viewed as providing 5 hours of daily respite for the patient away from family pressures, expectations and tensions. It also seeks to ease the deep-seated emotions that accompany the disease and which may be partially responsible for some of the unacceptable behavior often displayed at home. In this program, expectations are realistic and patients are supported at whatever level they can function. The program gears its expectations for success.

Our patients have often exceeded our limited expectations. For example, prior to opening the program for client participation, we conducted extensive staff education for all departments and center employees. In training the food-services staff, we anticipated that our patient group would have to be served food that was already cut up and that many patients would have to be fed. This expectation was based on family reports and research. Therefore, we prepared the staff accordingly. The very first day of the program, we brought the patients to the dining room to orient them to the setting and the food service. Without further direction, the patients picked up trays, cafeteria-style, chose the foods they wanted and proceeded to carry their own trays to the table. They chose their table mates, cut their own food, fed themselves, and even bussed their own tables. This came as a complete surprise to the staff and especially to the family caregivers. Mealtime became one of the more effective and enjoyable socializing experiences of the program. We quickly learned (a) that patients may often be capable of more than we expect and (b) to try self-care first, before "doing for" the patient.

An additional goal of the program was to try to effect some changes in the various difficult home situations by helping the caregivers to correct some of the confused communication and inappropriate expectations. Therefore, an important dimension was the nature and goals of family involvement in a psycho-educational component. This became one of the major features of the program.

To ensure this dimension of the plan, part of our contract with the family required that each family caregiver give 1 day a week to the program to act as volunteer-assistant with a patient other than their enrolled relative. Thus the program secured much-needed extra eyes and hands, while at the same time providing a teaching/learning experience for the family. This was accompanied by a range of formal and informal opportunities for interpretation and explanation of the program, its goals, processes and purposes, as well as monthly family meetings and individual conferences with the caregivers.

For the caring person this program provides the following benefits:
1. A laboratory for gaining a better understanding of the course of

the illness and for learning some techniques that may be used in daily interactions with the patient at home.

2. A demonstration of some of the methods of suitable communication and some ways of working with and helping the patient.

3. By working with a patient other than their own relative (while at the same time being in a position to observe their relative), family members expanded their understanding of the illness and its effects upon individuals.

4. It provides opportunities for respite to the caregivers.

5. When it became necessary, individualized planning and preparation for another living and care arrangement was begun early with the help of professional staff and in a supportive, nonthreatening, nonjudgmental environment.

I can offer no more appropriate summary of the value of this program to patient and family than to conclude with the following unsolicited letter that we received from the daughter of one of our patients:

Dear Dr. Saul,

I would like to share some thoughts and observations with you as to the progress of my mother, a patient in your group for 6 months now.

When you interviewed my mother at the end of March, you expressed that you believed she was advanced and that I should expect no cures or miracles. I agreed with your diagnosis because I have lived with her almost 7 years now and I am her sole caring person. I have watched her decline to the point where she no longer recognized me and every room in the house became strange to her. She was unresponsive, closed-up, something very close to a zombie. It's as if she were in a coma with her eyes open.

She started in your group in May and the change in her is nothing short of miraculous. She has become a social butterfly, responsive, eager to participate, helpful to the other patients and a changed person at home. When I speak to her, she becomes alert and answers me. It's not always the answer I expect or want, but she answers me!

Her very first day in your group was a milestone in our house. She came home and said nothing—but that night at dinner (almost 6 hours after she came home) she said, "We had so much fun today—all we did was laugh. I played ball and had a good time. I even danced." This was the first sentence she completed in more than a year and it was about something that happened hours earlier. My teenage son and I were amazed.

Neighbors notice how sociable she is now—she waves and smiles and says she's fine when asked.

In my opinion, had she never been exposed to your group she would have shrivelled and declined so severely by now that she would probably be bedridden. Your group is keeping her alive physically, mentally and psychologically. She is thriving on it. It is vital that she be there everyday and I schedule all her appointments so she will not miss a session.

To be perfectly honest with you, I originally thought of this group as a blessing for me—a relief from the "36-hour day" but after observing her change, I realize that it is way beyond that and how vital it is to her well-being.

Well, so many words to say simply—bless you, bless your loving and caring staff and bless the work you are doing.

Can there possibly be a better, more positive evaluation for this program?

Caregiver Concerns

16

Who Cares for the Caregiver? The History of Women in Caregiving

Sandra Lewenson, EdD, RN

Most caregivers needing respite care are women (Bader 1985; Hooyman, La Russo, Matthews and Nichols 1986; Miller 1985; Montgomery 1986). They provide care for families, for friends and for strangers. Typically, women find themselves in what is known as the "sandwich" generation. Caught between their children leaving home and the increasing disabilities of their aging parents they often give up career, personal time and private lives to care for an elderly family member. Moreover, women live longer than men and provide care for their husbands. As a result of outliving their spouses, they often find themselves alone in the world when they themselves need care. Historically, women have had the caregiving role thrust upon them and it became accepted.

In this chapter, respite care refers to the myriad of relief services needed by the caregiver, ranging from companionship to skilled nursing care for the older person living at home. Since most caregiving in America is provided by women, this chapter addresses women's personal and professional roles and their historical relationship to respite care.

Caregiving and women's roles share a rich history that has recently come under study. Society has traditionally assumed that caring lies within the woman's natural domain, thus presumably an inherently known role that needed little outside education, training or support. One of the professional roles in which caring is essential is nursing. Historically, it was believed that nurses needed little, if any, education to nurse. Just as it was assumed that nursing was a natural role, it is assumed today that caregiving is a natural role. The result of such thinking is reflected in the fact that there are too few respite care programs for caregivers, too little money to support such programs and too little training for the caregiver. The caregiver and those who relieve the caregiver—homemakers, home health aides and registered nurses—are hostages in a health care system that refuses to prioritize caregiving. Low priority means inadequate funding for respite care programs. The stigma society places on this role has led contemporary historian Susan Reverby (1987) to write that society does not value caring. Not only does the caregiver suffer from society's false assumptions, but our ever increasing older population suffers as well.

In order to understand the challenges respite care faces today, one can look at the history of American nursing. The nursing profession, still comprised of over 97 percent women, shares a common heritage with the woman's caregiving role. The growth of the nursing profession traces the historical route of caregiving in America. We see the dilemmas women have faced—first as untrained caregivers and later as trained nurses—observing insufficient political support, public interest and funding for nursing and for respite care. Furthermore, both share in the bias society shows when allocating health care dollars—supporting expensive technology rather than paying for long-term respite programs. Although both are important in a healthy society, better understanding of the latter is sorely needed. Thus, it is important to understand the background of caregiving and women's work in relation to today's concept of respite care.

Prior to 1873 and the opening of nurse training schools in America, women provided nursing care in the home. Women cooked, cleaned, changed linen, lowered fevers and nurtured their families. Historian Gerda Lerner, in her book *The Female Experience*, included the nineteenth-century diary of an Ohio farm women, Marian Louise Moore. The following passage reflects Moore's experience and feelings about nursing her 97-year-old mother in the spring of 1872. In this piece the 59-year-old Marian Louise Moore tells how she cooked, cleaned and worked at farming chores while providing care for her mother. We see her struggle with guilt when she was called away for a short time and had no one to assist her in caring for her mother.

I fear I was the transgressor on my beloved Mother's health....My Mother now being in the ninety-seventh year of her age bid fair to have lived four or five years longer for ought I could see...if she could have the proper indulgence and peace her age required....In the Spring of 1872...she was sick three months, part of the time helpless, typhoid inflammatory rheumatism.... This sickness of hers brought more work upon me, washing and other work, when I had more work of my own than I could possibly do....I was asked if I understood giving her medicine. I did but I did not understand performing all the unusual labor I did with a sick patient on my hands. Not a teaspoon was placed to her lips or work done for her but what I done (Lerner 1977).

Marian Louise Moore continued her work on the farm—painting the house, washing windows, harvesting barrels of apples—all the while caring for her mother. Often she had to leave her alone while she ran errands in the village and she recalls one time when she returned home and found her mother in a cold house because the fire had burned down in her absence. She told her, "Mother you have taken cold, and I won't leave you again."

Women traditionally have provided health care in their families and communities, learning this role by apprenticeship and experience. However, in 1873, nurse training schools began to open in American hospitals, signifying the first time that women formally studied the nursing role. Influenced by the work of Florence Nightingale, these schools looked to women to take charge of nurses' training and launched what became known as the modern nursing movement. More than simply following medical orders, nursing developed its own prescriptions for care. Trained nurses instituted sanitary reforms providing patients with pure air, clean linens, healthy foods and airy rooms that were well ventilated and bright with sunshine. The importance of clean, sanitary and restful environments was taught in accordance with Florence Nightingale's classic nursing text, *Notes on Nursing*, published in 1858 (Kalisch and Kalisch 1986; Nightingale 1969).

Hospitals recognized that a nurse training program provided them with a cheap labor force. Student nurses provided the nursing care at hospitals, while new graduates of training schools looked elsewhere for jobs. Those new graduates became independent nurses and worked as private duty nurses for families who could afford their fees. In order to find jobs, private duty nurses signed up at nursing registries opened by doctors, hospitals and some training school alumnae associations. Such agencies referred private duty nurses to families who requested their services. In this way, families could be relieved of the burdens and demands of providing care for a sick or elderly family member. The professionally trained nurse gave families rest and support (Birnbach and Lewenson 1991; Kalisch and Kalisch 1986; Lewenson 1992).

In the late nineteenth and early twentieth century, social reforms such as the public health movement led to the development of public health nursing. The public health nurse offered skilled caregiving services to the working-class family who could rarely pay for the private duty nurse. Lillian Wald (1867-1940), considered to be one of the first public health nurses, began the Henry Street Settlement on the Lower East Side in New York City. She provided nursing services to low-income families starting with nine nurses in 1893 and increasing the number to over 250 by 1916. Graduates from nurse training schools became the public health nurses who lived at the settlement house on Henry Street. They provided health care services to the underserved immigrant population. Public health nurses at Henry Street, and at new voluntary agencies that were springing up across the country, dressed wounds, lowered fevers, taught mothers to care for children, comforted the elderly and relieved families of total health care responsibilities. In essence they provided home care and respite for families in their community.

During America's industrialization, family structures and roles changed as families moved into cities to find jobs. Women stayed home caring for the family as men worked outside the home in the newly created jobs. Some women were attracted to the late nineteenth-century woman's movement and challenged established women's roles. They looked to colleges for an education and found jobs in a newly opening labor market. Women entered teaching, medicine, nursing and industry and found not only a new role but new financial independence as well.

At the same time, hospitals, following the opening of nurse training schools, became safer places for families to rely on for needed health care. Scientific discoveries, the advancement of the medical profession and the sanitary reforms instituted by trained nurses all contributed to an ever increasing trust in the American hospital. Nurse training schools provided women with training opportunities for financial independence and a new way of life. Hospitals also began to offer a safe environment in which families could place their loved ones for care, thus freeing the family from the sole burden of caregiving.

However, the path of professional nursing, in hospitals and in communities, confronted obstacles from those who did not believe nurses needed to control their own practice or provide for their own education. Nurses faced controls set by those outside the profession, which politically limited the type of nursing care services they could provide, fostered low pay by hospital employers and encouraged out-moded apprenticeship training. As a result, nursing's image shifted from one that attracted the "new educated independent woman" of the late nineteenth-century, to one that attracted women into a seemingly sub-servient "trained" role.

As we approach a new century, the role and image of the profes-sional registered nurse continues to be challenged. Higher education for nurses is essential to prepare practitioners able to provide complex caregiving services to an aging and more acutely ill population. Families need someone to whom they can turn to help them care for an aging parent—to learn simple caregiving methods, to give medications correctly and to help plan a respite from their own exhaustive caregiving. As professional caregivers, registered nurses provide such health care services assisting families in achieving higher levels of health. Paraprofessionals, including homemakers and home health aides, provide hours of respite for those needing physical care and companionship. Caregivers can receive time off to work and rest when such respite care is available. However, whether one is an untrained caregiver, a paraprofessional or a registered professional nurse, all share in society's assumption that caregiving is a women's "natural" role, needing little if any education or support. Despite the teaching, emotional support and physical relief these workers offer to caregivers, each one experiences the stigma of low pay, little advancement and the low status of their work.

The literature tells us that most elderly "patients" requiring respite care are women. As women they experience additional negative consequences from an ageist and sexist society. Moreover, these patients often need total 24-hour physical and emotional care as a result of debilitating conditions such as rheumatoid arthritis, stroke or Alzheimer's disease. Family members caring for elderly patients are more likely to be women than men (Bader 1985). Women who care for their husbands and parents alter their work and living arrangements to do so. When men provide caregiving services, they experience the same attitudes as women do, receiving little financial or emotional support from others.

A review of society's historical responses to care and caregiving roles informs us today about how we want to plan for care in the future. In a society that values caring, we should know the pain and fear that caregivers feel when they are vulnerable and alone. We should rank respite care as important and should assure that no one is left exposed and unembraced. In doing so we will be better able to provide the help caregivers have been asking for ever since the days of Marian Louise Moore.

REFERENCES

Bader, J. Respite care: temporary relief for caregivers. *Women and Health* 10(2/3): 39-52, 1985.

Birnbach, N. and S. Lewenson, eds. *First Words: Selected Addresses from the National League for Nursing, 1894-1933*. New York: National League for Nursing Press, 1991.

Hooyman, N., M. LaRusso, M. Matthews and J. Nichols. The Caregiver's Perspective. In R. Montgomery and J. Prothero, eds., *Developing Respite Services for the Elderly*. Seattle: University of Washington Press, 1986.

Kalisch P. and B. Kalisch. *The Advance of American Nursing, 2nd Ed.* Boston: Little, Brown, 1986.

Lerner, G. Nursing and the Aged Mother. In *The Female Experience: An American Documentary*. Indianapolis: Bobbs-Merrill, 1977.

Lewenson, S. *Taking Charge: Nursing, Suffrage, and Feminism in America, 1873-1920.* New York: Garland, 1992.

Lewis, M. Older women and health: an overview. *Women and Health* 10(2/3):1-16, 1977.

McKelvey, R. Wounded nature. *JAMA* 265(23):3183, 1991.

Miller, D. Women and long-term nursing care. *Women and Health* 10(2/3):29-38, 1985.

Montgomery, R. Researching Respite: Beliefs, Facts and Questions. In R. Montgomery and J. Prothero, eds., *Developing Respite Services for the Elderly*. Seattle: University of Washington Press, 1986.

Nightingale, F. *Notes on Nursing* (1858). New York: Dover, 1969.

Reverby, S. *Ordered to Care: The Dilemma of American Nursing, 1850-1945.* Cambridge: Cambridge University Press, 1987.

17

The Caregiver:
The Forgotten Patient

Carlo E. Grossi, MD and Parathasarthy Narasinham, MD

The stress of taking care of patients with advanced cancer and terminal illness can often result in burnout of both professional staff and family caregivers. Often these individuals are the "forgotten patients," the victims of significant continuous stress both at the hospital and at home. The aim of this chapter is to address their needs and offer a plan to help them resolve the problem of burnout and offer respite care to the forgotten patient.

Burnout has long been recognized in intensive care unit nurses and physicians. It is characterized by feelings of depression, hopelessness and loss of drive and optimism in trying to help critically ill patients. Similarly, staff working in oncology units who are involved in giving complex chemotherapy regimens to very sick patients will become discouraged if they see repeated failures and high mortality. One must understand that if one takes care of terminally ill patients there is a need for respite from the constant stress. The means used to resolve this problem may be different for the health worker than for the family caregiver at home. In addition to the stress of a terminal illness, the lay home caregiver has a close emotional attachment to the patient and little understanding of the medical process involved.

Burnout in oncology units and large tumor clinics is an established syndrome and it requires recognition and treatment by staff as well as the medical resources of the institution. Burnout experienced by the lay caregiver of a family member or friend is a similar syndrome but requires a different solution using hospice and available medicosocial and community resources.

Burnout of the professional caregiver occurs in both hospital and clinic settings. The constant stress of taking care of very ill patients with advanced cancer and of young adults and children with leukemia or sarcomas can result in feelings of hopelessness and despair. The chances of response are small and with young patients, the caregivers may identify with the patient or the family. They may be deeply affected by the deterioration and death of the patient. This may be interpreted as a failure of the medical protocol and their expertise. In a busy hospital burnout may not be easily recognized at first. Sometimes the person in charge of the oncology unit has such a big ego that he refuses to admit that such a syndrome is possible in his team. Fatigue and insomnia may be looked upon as a sign of weakness rather than evidence of slow burnout. It is very important that such individuals be offered help and given respite care.

Respite care can be provided by offering a temporary change of assignments, taking more time off for recreation, or attending medical conferences related to the work being done. The latter permits the health worker to meet and communicate with other peers on this topic and see how they deal with it. Group discussions between medical and nursing staff may be too close and personal to be effective. It must be realized that many of these physicians, nurses and social workers already attend family support group sessions and bereavement group meetings themselves. They may also benefit from a change in environment by attending meetings outside the hospital and outside the city. By attending meetings elsewhere they become aware that others have similar problems and they have a chance to compare notes with peers from other institutions. They can then see that in spite of medical advances in multidisciplinary care, the benefit is not yet great. In addition the caregiver should seek the help of a professional counselor such as a clinical psychologist or a psychiatrist who is familiar with these issues. This can be of great help in formulating long-range adjustments to a very demanding profession. It will also help the health worker to return to work with realistic expectations and a better ability to deal with the stress of terminal illness.

Burnout of the family caregiver creates an even greater need for respite care. Once the patient goes to a hospice or dies, the family caregiver becomes indeed the "forgotten patient." The family caregiver tries to give as much physical and emotional support as possible to the patient at home, usually with little help from the community. One must realize that once a patient with a terminal illness such as cancer goes home there will likely be only a short semiweekly visit from the nurse, some help from a health aide and an occasional call from the physician. The rest of the time the family members are the total caregivers for control of pain and assisting the bedridden patient with body functions. This becomes extremely stressful even if there is a home companion. The breadwinner of the family has to work during the day and try to take care of a spouse or elderly parent at night. There is need for continuing support of the caregiver at home even though prospective plans were made at the hospital. Visits by a social worker, or a clinical nurse specialist or the family doctor can help meet the stress of the illness. However, this is not enough and some physical relief must be offered on a regular basis. In this setting it is essential that respite be offered so that the caregiver can get some sleep and attend to outside activities other than work. One option is certain forms of hospice care that can offer needed respite to the family or friend taking care of the moribund patient with cancer.

In New York City there is a hospice at the Cabrini Medical Center that has provided this needed form of respite for the caregiver at home. The patient is admitted to the hospice for 3 to 4 days so that the family can have relief and some time off and be able to attend to necessary business and social functions. This allows the caregiver to resume some normal activity without feeling guilty, and knowing that the loved one is receiving expert medical and nursing care. This also allows the medical staff to reformulate pain regimen schedules and to address nutritional needs and any necessary change in medications. The patient can then return home aware that the hospice has helped him and is involved in the supervision of his medical care. The family has received respite care as well. In smaller communities where there are only two or three hospitals, the clinical oncology community program and American Cancer Society volunteers often coordinate the care of the hospital hospice program. In a very large city there are many elderly cancer patients with no relatives and few friends. Here the hospice concept is harder to work out. The need for a terminal care hospital has become evident. In New York City, Calvary Hospital was established to fulfill this need for the terminally ill. For the last 20 years this hospital, under the support of the Catholic Archdiocese of New York, has offered care to patients in their last months of life. This has allowed caregivers at home to be able to get help for their loved ones in the final days of their illness and also to have respite and prepare for the loss and bereavement. The presence of experienced nurses, social workers and physicians has permitted caregivers to participate in support groups and accept with greater mental tranquility the inevitable death of their loved one.

Again the caregiver remains the forgotten patient. All the focus of our resources is on the individual with terminal illness and it is assumed that the lay caregiver will stay well. To help the caregiver there are family support groups that meet weekly in most oncology clinics and hospitals and bereavement groups that meet monthly. In our hospital family support groups, breast cancer groups and bereavement groups meet separately on a monthly basis. At these meetings there is a nurse oncology specialist, a social worker and an interested physician. These oncology support sessions are necessary to explain to the family the problems and complications of chemotherapy, surgery and radiotherapy. The breast survival group offers help in explaining the multimodal forms of cancer therapy being used and the need for screening mammography. This also allows the family member to better understand their course of treatment of the illness. The bereavement group meeting is the most important for the family to attend. Here they can ask the questions that they felt the doctor and the staff had not answered while the patient was alive. They can cope better with their loss by attending these meetings. By meeting others that have had a similar tragedy they can share their grief and their recovery. This group therapy has been most successful in our hospital in giving the "forgotten patient" counseling and help. It has permitted a more rapid readjustment and return to the mainstream of daily activities.

The need for respite care is urgent for both the health professional with burnout or the lay caregiver at home. For the health professional, time off, temporary change of assignments, group conferences and professional counseling have been of help. In severe cases psychiatric help may be needed. For the lay family caregiver respite care for the forgotten patient can take several forms. If hospice is available, use of its facilities on a temporary basis can provide relief from the extreme pressures and stress of a terminal illness at home. Adult day care, described in depth in Chapter 5 is another alternative. When these options are not available, a terminal care hospital is advised before the caregiver breaks down. In addition the caregiver should seek help through support groups or by individual counseling by a psychiatric social worker or clinical psychologist. It is the responsibility of the treating physician and oncology unit that has coordinated the care at home to guard against the breakdown of the home caregiver by providing organized help and advice.

18

Caregiver Stress
and Respite Care

Maura Ryan, PhD, RNC, GNP

An epidemic exists in the United States today. What was until recent decades episodic and not a particularly widespread problem has now broken upon the national health care consciousness with great impact; this epidemic is *caregiver* stress.

The changing demographics of our society, in which people are living longer, pave the way for the increasing incidence of chronic ailments, impaired ability for self-care and, because of recent medical advances, a longer survival time. As the needs of the frail elderly increase, so also do the demands on those who are responsible for their care. Only a small percentage of those over 65 reside in nursing homes and the remainder of those who are disabled are cared for in the community. Although some elderly require no care in order to function independently, many American seniors are dependent for care on others and without this help they would require institutionalization.

It is well documented in the literature (e.g., Shanas 1979; Brody 1981) that families are committed to caring for their elderly family members at home, frequently at tremendous emotional, physical and financial cost. Even beyond the point where a substantial toll has already been wrought, most families have no choice but to provide care to their elderly relatives and at the same time to carry on with their already hectic life styles. This results in varying degrees of stress, also referred to as caregiver burden, strain or burnout (Baldwin 1990).

Trying to determine or to predict the factors that are associated with caregiver stress and strain are infinitely complex. According to Elaine Brody (1990), not only do "different caregivers experience different amounts and kinds of strains, but the various factors that produce strain interact with each other in intricate ways." These stresses are not just of the variety associated with providing hands-on care that may be physically exhausting, time-consuming and not in any way to be underestimated, but they also entail complex interplays between parent and child, mother and daughter and mother-in-law/daughter-in-law, whose patterns of interacting was established long before the caregiving started.

The term "caregiver" can cover a broad range of activities depending on a person's degree of disability, physical proximity, financial status and living arrangements. Inherent in the role of caregiver is a sense of parenting except that the type of relationship can differs. Adult children expect their own children whom they care for to grow up to attain independence, while elderly care recipients, in contrast, grow frailer and more dependent. What may start out as an occasional task can progress over the course of months or years to 24-hour direct care. Horowitz (1985) identified four broad categories of caregiving behavior: (1) direct hands-on care (functional care), such as assisting with bathing, dressing, feeding, getting out of bed, moving in and out doors, administering medication and taking care of shopping, banking and general housework; (2) emotional support; (3) financial assistance and (4) mediating with formal organizations such as governmental, social and health care agencies.

Approximately 75 percent of caregivers are female. Women have traditionally been the primary caregivers of young children. As our society lives longer they have been placed back in the caregiver role. Family well-being has historically been a female activity and until recent decades, this has been a woman's primary function. Unmarried daughters, if they exist, do not usually reside with parents and therefore no longer automatically inherit the caregiver role. Nowadays the primary caregiver is more likely to be an elderly spouse; approximately 50 percent of caregivers are elderly females who simultaneously must confront their own aging, lack of stamina and multiple health problems. The added stress of being responsible for someone else's care and well-being also places them in a vulnerable position. As a matter of fact the caretaker is sometimes referred to as the silent patient.

Adult daughters (married or single but living in a separate residence), daughters-in-law, nieces, friends and sons comprise, in that order, the remaining caregiver cohort. No doubt many readers of this chapter are responsible for the care of an elderly relative. Contemporary literature now refers to female offspring who are now caregivers to their parent as members of "the sandwich generation" or "women in the middle." Not only are they middle-aged developmentally, but they are caught in the middle between the demands of their aging parents, their own children, their spouses and their careers. The Older Womens' League, in their 1989 *Mother's Day Report*, estimated that today's women will spend an average of 17 years caring for their own children and 18 years in caring for their parents and they foresee the day when American couples will spend more time caring for their parents than for their children.

There are many positive benefits that can be derived from caring for older parents; among them are feelings of satisfaction for fulfilling societal roles, conforming to religious or cultural expectations, repaying parents for their upbringing, expressing affection and providing a good role model for their children in anticipation of their own later years (Brody 1990). Nevertheless, there are many consequences that have a negative effect on emotional well-being, physical health, life style and financial status. Emotional stress has been identified as the single most severe and negative consequence of caregiving.

Many symptoms resulting from caregiving have been identified. They include physical illnesses such as ulcers, high blood pressure, weight loss or weight gain, asthma and eczema. In the emotional realm, feelings of alienation, hostility, anger, fatigue, helplessness, hopelessness, social isolation, loneliness, anxiety, victimization, aggression, powerlessness, frustration, guilt, sleeplessness, irritability, lowered morale, depression, personal neglect and emotional exhaustion have been reported by approximately half of all caregivers. A rather startling finding by Kielcott-Glazer (1987) indicated that caregivers have poorer immune function than their age-matched peers and this predisposes them to increased risk of infection.

In addition, caregivers report restrictions on their time, freedom, relationships, social and recreational activities, privacy and space when an older person actually moves into the household. Caregiving of an elderly person can result in strained or shattered marriages, rebellions on the part of offspring and less discretionary income, because caregivers spend varying amounts of income on the care recipients. Conflicting demands and difficulties in setting priorities are also problematic. If siblings have unresolved feelings of anger or resentment toward the now feeble parent because he or she had not been an "ideal" parent or because the parent was abusive toward them as children, then the stage is set for numerous intergenerational conflicts including, in some instances some form of elder abuse. Caregiving has a ripple effect that has personal, familial and workplace implications.

Caregivers are not the only ones that experience negative feelings or stress reactions in this situation. Care recipients also suffer because they must forfeit their independence; they have to admit that they are no longer able to take care of themselves and that they are getting old and feeble. They fear becoming a burden and feel guilty for imposing on their families. Unresolved conflicts between parent and offspring may now intensify—the shoe is on the now other foot.

Ironically, the care recipients' attempts to remain independent and care for themselves when they are no longer capable of doing so becomes yet another source of stress to the caregiver. Family caregivers have many needs regarding stress reduction. Curiously, however, there is documented *under-utilization* of most available services by many caregivers. In 1987, the Alzheimer's Disease and Related Disorders Association polled the readers of its newsletter to identify their most pressing needs. Respite care, formal community-based care and financial support were the areas most frequently identified, with over 50 percent citing overnight respite care as a high priority. According to Fortinsky and Hathaway (1990), present challenges in elder care are twofold: (1) to link caregivers with available services in order to preserve their own health and well-being, and (2) to continue to develop appropriate services for caregivers as well as care recipients. In support of the first challenge, health care professionals have a responsibility to encourage caregivers to care for themselves because they cannot effectively care for others unless they care for themselves first. This agenda is particularly crucial for those who care for those suffering from the organic brain syndromes including Alzheimer's disease, not only because of the complexity of the condition, but because survival time from diagnosis to demise can be as long as 20 years. Moreover, caretaking for these types of people often becomes the lot of a caretaker spouse who is generally also frail and has multiple chronic health problems.

Respite care has been identified as the single most important service that can be provided to families (Baldwin 1990). It is unique in that it provides services to those who care as well as to those who receive care. It provides a wide range of services; it can be delivered in a variety of settings, including the home, and is based on the physical and psychological needs of the consumer as well as convenience, availability and cost of the service (Looney 1987). Considering the fact that the potential for institutionalization increases with advancing age, that caregivers experience more severe overall problems and greater stress levels than the general population, and that respite care is considerably less expensive than institutionalization, it is surprising that it is still underutilized. Some linkage is missing between the identified need and the utilization of services.

Adult day care programs as a source of support and respite number over 2000 nationally and are probably the most utilized of all the respite programs. Nurses and social workers who are employed in such settings have an ideal opportunity to reach caregivers and to impart some practical suggestions for building "stress busters" into their daily routine and for instituting support groups, conducting workshops, making books, pamphlets, video tapes and community/state resource lists available to caregivers.

Beverly Baldwin, a nurse researcher who has written extensively on caregiver issues, has suggested the following stress reduction techniques:

1. Taking one day at a time
2. Using positive self-talk
3. Practicing visualization, meditation, deep breathing and regular physical exercise

She also suggests:

4. Avoiding overreactions to troublesome situations
5. Setting goals
6. Recognizing that present family relationships cannot be erased
7. Identifying the most stressful activities, the type, the time of day and the frequency of occurrences and then to try to plan strategies to deal with them
8. Being kind to yourself, giving yourself rewards, taking mini-breaks such as a hot bubble bath, and practicing yoga or meditation
9. Keeping your sense of humor—when all else fails it's a definite stress buster!

REFERENCES

Baldwin, B. Family caregiving: trends and forecast. *Geriatric Nursing* 10:172-175, 1990.

Brody, E. Women in the middle and family help to old people. *Gerontologist* 21(5):471-480, 1981.

Fortinsky, R. and T. Hathaway. Information and service needs among active and former family caregivers of persons with Alzheimer's disease. *Gerontologist* 30(5):604-609, 1990.

Horowitz, A. Sons and daughters as caregivers to older parents: differences in role performance and consequences. *Gerontologist* 25:612-617, 1985.

Kielcott-Glazer, J., et al. Chronic stress and immunity in family caregivers of Alzheimer's disease victims. *Psychosomatic Med.* 49:523-535, 1987.

Looney, K. The respite care alternative. *J. Gerontol. Nursing* 13(5):18-23, 1987.

Older Women's League. Failing America's caregivers: a status report on women
    who care. *Mother's Day Report,* 1987.
Shanas, E. Social myth as hypothesis: the case of the family relations of old people.
    Gerontologist 19:3-9, 1979.

19

A Life-style Rehabilitation Approach to Manage the Stress of Caregiving

Lynn M. Tepper, EdD

Life is challenging, from the moment of birth to the moment of death. Throughout our lives, each and every one of us is confronted repeatedly with problems and challenges. During these difficult times, it is comforting to know that we do possess the skills and resources that will help us make the best of difficult situations.

A wealth of information has been collected by researchers on how people cope with life's challenges. Many of these approaches have been popularized in magazines and television and radio talk shows and they have also been incorporated into community-based self-help programs. Large corporations use consultants to present "stress management" seminars for their employees; the military requires staff to attend stress management courses; some hospitals offer community-based workshops on stress management, often with an emphasis on coping with chronic, debilitating illness; colleges and universities have recently begun to offer formal stress management courses to their students. The self-help movement of the 1970s created hundreds of support groups which, among other things, had the underlying purpose of assisting with stresses that result from some of life's most demanding roles, conditions and afflictions. I have spent the past 10 years teaching stress management to both undergraduate and graduate students, with an emphasis on assessment of one's own stress-proneness, and the management of some of the stresses inherent to this population. My concern as a gerontologist however, is why stress management is so rarely applied to a group of people who are under one of the most extreme conditions of stress—caregivers. This population consists mainly of two groups: the *formal* caregivers, employed by institutions, agencies and individuals to provide care to the frail, terminally ill, dying or otherwise severely impaired patient, and the *informal* caregivers, who are mostly friends and family, who provide a similar level of care for the same type of afflicted individuals. Experience with these two types of caregivers has shown that the latter group—families and friends—encounters a slightly different kind of stress *in addition* to the stresses also experienced by the first group—the stress of providing care to someone they are emotionally attached to, someone whom they knew when they were well and vital, whom they are not being paid to care for, and for whom they have already begun to grieve for.

Few other conditions place so much stress on family members and friends as caregiving. Caregivers routinely report stress-related symptoms such as depression, anxiety, hostility and fatigue. They are often angry or resentful and feel guilty about not doing enough. The stresses they experience originate from many sources, such as housekeeping, dressing, feeding, toileting and keeping vigilant watch over the patient, and perhaps dealing with behavioral changes and disturbances—an experience that can be particularly painful. Moreover, caregivers often experience a great sense of psychological and personal loss as they see their relative or friend gradually decline. Often the care they provide demands all or almost all of their time. Perhaps they may even be criticized by other relatives or friends. They usually get little relief or respite from the daily stress they encounter. Because social support may be often be lacking, there is rarely anyone to articulate an accurate understanding of the caregiver's experience. There is a tendency for caregivers to become isolated, and this decrease in social contact may be the single most stressful element in caregiving.

Respite can provide the "pause" necessary to refresh and replenish and those that take part in respite programs are sometimes better caregivers than those who do not. However, *all* caregivers are in desperate need of managing the stresses inherent to caregiving, and *all* caregivers do have the capacity to reduce this stress by employing some "tried and true" approaches that have been known to work.

The good news is that as human beings we are adaptable. Our ability to cope is not fixed at birth. We develop it and perfect it throughout our lives, either consciously or unconsciously. We need not be passive bystanders. Knowledge is power and empowerment will certainly assist us all to gain a greater sense of control over the challenges of our lives.

Over the years, I have read volumes of material dealing with the topic of stress management. These books, journals, articles and scientific reports focus almost entirely on the following topics: defining stress, learning how to cope, building a support system, self-assessment of stress, problem-solving, relaxation techniques, maintaining internal control, self-talk, developing a sense of humor, self-reward, avoidance, having realistic expectations and thinking adaptive thoughts. These are certainly important aids in the management of stress, but they are sorely lacking in their ability to help us focus on our need to "rehabilitate" our life style in ways that will not only make us feel better and fortify us with the strength necessary to deal with the stresses we are experiencing, but provide us with "habits" that will keep us healthier and perhaps add some years to our lives as well as some life to our years.

The approaches I am referring to are sleep, exercise and nutrition. These are the energizing or fortifying approaches to managing stress, especially the kinds of stresses that we more or less have to live with and that are not easily avoidable.

Sleep, exercise and nutrition come under the category of an approach we can call "building resistance." We know that both the physiology and the psychology of stress often result in exhaustion. This occurs because the body's reserves of energy, both physiologic and psychic, have been drawn down too low. Exhaustion, we also know, places one in a more vulnerable position for illness. This knowledge suggests that an important principle for stress management and control is the following: *The stronger the body's reserves, the better able the body will be to resist the ravages of stress.* How do you strengthen your body's reserves? The answer is by considering three factors: sleep, exercise and nutrition.

SLEEP

Research tells us that the brain needs to rest in order to maintain its equilibrium. When sleep is too brief, too fitful or disrupted, we awaken irritable, tired, cranky and less able to cope. This is because the biochemical and electrical balances are not maintained. We see a range of problems that result from mild to severe sleep disturbances. The chronic, long-term disturbances cause physical and psychological exhaustion, depression and high levels of anxiety. In this regard rapid-eye-movement, or REM, is very important. REM sleep is the stage of the sleep cycle when dreams occur, and dream completion is vital for psychological well-being. If awakened during this stage of sleep, we may experience mood swings, depression, irritability, distractibility and difficulty concentrating. Sleep, then, must have four qualities: it must be full, relaxed, continuous and long enough. Although it is true that as we age we require less sleep, research shows that most of us need 6 to 8 hours in order to function optimally the next day. What factors influence the quality of our sleep? Among them are the degree of relaxation vs. tension in our lives, what we ate before sleeping, what we did physically, the events of the following day, what we've done to resolve conflicts, the bed and the room temperature, and the environment of the sleeping room. Below are some suggestions for improving the quality of sleep.

Food Consumption

There are four basic rules concerning consumption of food before going to bed:

1. Don't overeat at dinner (a small dinner is preferable)
2. Avoid late evening snacks, especially coffee, chocolate and foods that are high in sugar
3. Limit fluid intake 2 to 3 hours before retiring
4. Limit alcoholic beverages at night (except wine, which is all right in moderation)

The Environment

Suggestions related to the sleep environment include the following:

1. Sleep in a place supportive of sleep
2. Sleep on a firm mattress
3. Sleep in a quiet place; try to avoid noise from loud neighbors, clocks, barking dogs, and from the street
4. Oil a creaky bed frame
5. Use dark window shades or drapes if you are sensitive to light
6. Avoid sleeping in extreme temperatures (65 to 68 degrees is usually about right)

Attitudes

The sleeper's attitude upon retiring is also important.

1. Accept sleep as a normal, desirable event
2. Don't ruminate about unfinished business
3. Approach bedtime with a positive attitude: a feeling of "closure" and a positive feeling about the following day
4. It's easier to fall asleep when you are psychologically and physically ready; flow with your mood, and don't force yourself to sleep if you're not tired (a warm bath or reading can sometimes be helpful)

5. A relaxing routine before going to bed will make you feel calmer and will help you feel ready to go to sleep

Relaxing Routines

It is useful to develop before-bed routines that are calming, like taking a warm bath, having a small glass of warm milk, or having a quiet talk with your spouse or roommate. Some people read relaxing material, meditate, do deep breathing exercises, practice deep muscle relaxation, employ autogenic training or visualize something positive about the next day. Television programs or reading materials that are too stimulating or frightening should be avoided.

Rest

Rest is important during the daytime. Research supports the fact that those who have rest periods during the day have far fewer illnesses. Rest periods should be used wisely, and should be of high quality. A "rest" that consists of a cup of coffee, a jelly donut and a cigarette usually results in just the opposite effect. I suggest a change in environment—try a quiet place, where there are few people around. Regular periods of rest should become a part of your life style.

EXERCISE

Exercise can be as valuable to the body as sleep and rest are to the brain. Research confirms that a high level of physical arousal results in the release of tension and restores energy reserves. When people are physically fit they can actually reduce or prevent stress and disease. Exercise consists of a wide range of physical acts, ranging from cardiovascular conditioning, respiratory conditioning and maintaining or increasing muscle tone, to taking a brisk walk on a regular basis.

Exercise has other benefits as well. It contributes to a better, more positive self-image and an attitude of control over one's life. Actually, whether or not we exercise may be determined by how much we like ourselves; clearly, we do not need to exercise to exist.

How do we know if we are physically fit? Listed below are some substantiated indications of *not* being fit.

1. Becoming short of breath after walking up a flight of stairs
2. A long recovery time after walking up a flight of stairs

3. A general feeling of exhaustion after a short period of physical exertion
4. Poor, fitful sleep
5. Depression, anxiety
6. General muscle tension
7. Obesity
8. Poor muscle tone; loose, flabby skin
9. Being winded after half an hour of tennis
10. Muscles cramped and aching after participating in sports
11. No energy left after a workday
12. General tiredness, fatigue, boredom
13. Frequent irritability
14. Little "joie de vivre"
15. Fear and discomfort with sensations under conditions of high arousal
16. Noticeable increase in heart rate after sex, anger, fright, physical strain or exercise
17. Inability to jog a mile in 8 minutes and recover breath within 5 minutes

The next step is to decide what kind of exercise you need. Several myths persist about exercise, such as, "Jogging is enough to get totally fit," "if you are over 60, don't strain" and "walking is enough." For every exercise known to man, there is an article stating why that exercise should not be used. Exercise has many purposes. It can improve flexibility, muscle tone and strength. It can relieve tension. It aids in weight control and reduction. With improved cardiovascular and respiratory functioning, more oxygen gets to the body's organs, including the brain. All of these things can enhance a person's ability to adapt to stress.

There are factors to consider when choosing an exercise, including entry level, age, level of fitness, history of exercise, active disease processes, physical structure and injuries. Carrying out a regimen of exercise is also important. The problem is that excuses can get in the way: "There's not enough time, it's boring, it's hard to get started, it's painful, I'm discouraged because I'm not losing weight," and so forth. There is another way to look at it: it took years to get out of shape, but it only takes a month to begin getting back in shape. Perhaps we should expect some discomfort initially. We should make exercise a habit, a commitment. Cost is a factor, and so is convenience. A good jump rope costs only about $10; greens fees can run into the thousands. Continuity is important, no matter what activity is chosen. Sedentary life styles are tough to break and old habits are easy to return to. Sharing an exercise activity with a friend or relative can create a built-in support system. If cardiovascular conditioning is your interest, it should be aerobic conditioning, if you are in good health. This will increase the capacity of your heart and lungs, and promote your body's use of oxygen. Aerobic exercise includes running, swimming, cycling, stair-climbing and fast-paced walking. Ultimately it is this cardiovascular conditioning that is part of a total stress-management approach. When you are fit, your body and mind can respond to and recover from stress reactions more readily. The type of exercise you choose should be done on a regular basis—three times per week and at least 20 minutes in duration. Doubling your heart rate should be a goal, but this depends on your age and medical approval. Aerobic conditioning stimulates a sense of well-being. It is based on cycles of arousal followed by relaxation. If your maximum heart rate is achieved, tension is released and relaxation can take place. Studies show that aerobic conditioning can lead to increased energy, a feeling of well-being, improved adaptability, decreased appetite, relief from sinus problems and shortened recovery times from stress reactions.

NUTRITION

Our body's reserves against stress can depend on diet. Unfortunately, eating habits start in childhood, so many of us may be at a slight disadvantage. To make matters worse, the guidelines we teach our children are often reflective of what we were taught during childhood. Another drawback is that we live in a society that emphasizes speedy food preparation in the home. These "fast foods" are usually highly processed, and high in salt and sugar. Some examples are partially precooked rice, white bread and canned vegetables. In addition, many people eat meals at fast food establishments because the cost is low and the wait is short. Consequently, many young people acquire bad eating habits and this results in an inability to conquer stress. Some of these habits include eating too fast and consuming too many calories. These bad habits are often followed by bloating, indigestion, discomfort and stress on the intestinal tract. Food may not be chewed well, so the stomach and intestines must work harder. When food contains too much fat, too many preservatives and too many by-products from processing, the stomach, gallbladder, liver, intestines and kidneys are overtaxed. Eating to excess is also a problem. Too much eating, smoking and drinking lessens our ability to manage stress and reduces our life expectancy. We have only to look at the long-lived populations of the world, such as the peoples of the Caucasus and Andes mountains, to see the benefits of sensible, healthy nutrition.

CONCLUSION

As human beings, we are exceptionally adaptable. We develop and perfect our repertoire of coping approaches during the entire course of our lives. We need not be passive bystanders. Knowledge is power, and empowerment will certainly assist us all to gain a greater sense of control over the challenges that life dictates. The personal decision to take part in a partial or total "life-style rehabilitation" is within our power and will assist us in the management of stress and tension.

Respite Care Research

20

The Vacation Needs of
Families with a Disabled Child

Joyce Storey, BSN, MSEd, RN

Families who care for a child with a disability in their home have become the focus of many social programs over the past two decades. These programs fall under the heading of family support services. Some of these services are more comprehensive and accessible than others. Trends in social programs prompted by federal legislation and a new emerging philosophy in education and human service fields encourage early intervention and family systems approaches to services (Dunst et al. 1988). One of these family support services is respite care. Respite care, defined by the Cerebral Palsy Associations as "a system of temporary supports for families and caregivers of developmentally disabled individuals which provides the family and caregiver with relief," has evolved in various forms. There is a need for further evolution in the development of respite care models of service that include a holistic, family systems approach.

This chapter proposes that models of respite care that provide for family leisure and recreation should not separate disabled children from their families. Family leisure and recreation need not and should not imply the absence of the disabled child; indeed, these activities can be made possible and further enhanced through the development of respite models that provide relief while keeping the family together. A vacation-type resort designed especially for these families is one model to be considered. This study seeks to establish the need for such models (as perceived by families and through a review of the existing literature) and to demonstrate that early intervention will strengthen families, enhance family functioning and promote the use of respite care in general.

STATEMENT OF THE PROBLEM

Although there appears to be much attention in the literature and from the government for supports to families in the form of respite, two recent national studies have made researchers painfully aware of the limitations in the delivery of respite services (Human Services Research Institute [HSRI] 1989, 1990). One type of respite care is the wide range of services for families who care for a child with a developmental disability or serious medical condition at home. Originally, this type of care was designed to give parents some relief, some respite, from the day-to-day demands of caring for a child with a disability. As it has evolved over the last decade, respite has come to mean any service or program that provides care for a person with a disability or the dependent elderly while the primary caregiver is engaged in some other activity. Under this expansive umbrella, all of the following situations can be found (HSRI 1989):

1. Beds in a mental retardation institution can be reserved periodically by parents. These same places are also available if a crisis arises that impairs the family's ability to care for its member with a disability.
2. Spaces in local group homes for people with disabilities can serve the same function as institutional programs.
3. A system whereby individual families take turns using respite facilities according to a preset schedule. Family members must confirm these dates at the beginning of the year or lose them.
4. A respite house or center—a group home serving exclusively as a respite facility—may often allow parents to schedule specific periods of respite, up to 2 full weeks, in advance. They also provide emergency respite so that a child living at home does not have to go into an institution during a family crisis.
5. A licensed respite provider will take a person with a disability into his or her home for any prearranged period of time ranging from a few hours to a week.
6. A respite agency will arrange for its employees to care for a person with a disability either in the family home or the provider's home.
7. A licensed practical nurse may be sent by a home health care agency on a weekly basis to provide respite for the parent of a severely disabled child so that the parent can perform necessary family chores, such as grocery shopping.
8. A regular day care center may accept children with disabilities.
9. A neighborhood center's after-school program may hire special

staff so that each of its activity groups can include one child with severe disabilities.

10. A neighbor, recruited and trained by the family itself, is certified by a state agency as a respite provider for that family.
11. A drop-in weekend day center with limited space may offer respite care for children with disabilities on a first-come, first-served basis.
12. A college student spends 3 hours every afternoon after school with a young man with autism, enabling both of his parents to retain their full-time jobs.

Listing all of these possibilities together creates the illusion that there is a comprehensive system of respite services that are sensitive to meeting any need a family may have. However, the reality is that in most areas families have few, if any, alternatives for securing useful respite care. If respite services do exist, they are likely to be limited to one or two possibilities and are presented to parents on a take-it-or-leave-it basis (HSRI 1989). For some parents the options presented are often not at all viable.

One important aspect of all the models listed and others (family cooperatives, camps and hotel rooms set aside for respite) is that they all separate the disabled child from his family. Because many of these families experience guilt when leaving their child with others, especially when they are leaving for the purpose of their own recreation, the absence of the child is often felt so strongly that the family cannot experience any real sense of leisure (CSR 1989; Devlin 1986; Green and Evans 1984; Robinson 1987; Salisbury and Intagliata 1986). Another risk is that wholesome family recreation and leisure, if realized, becomes associated with the absence of the disabled child and this is an unhealthy dynamic to establish and reinforce for parents and for well siblings. When taking a trip or even just having a weekend away means choosing between placing their disabled child in an institution or leaving him with a stranger, many parents will forego the trip (NICHEY 1989; HSRI 1989; Salisbury and Intagliata 1986; Ptacek et al. 1982; Upshur 1983).

HYPOTHESIS

Given the present selection and accessibility of respite care services, many families are never able to get the needed break—respite in the form of a vacation—that is so sorely needed by those in the seriously stressful position of constant in-home caregiving. Most families would take vacations if they could keep their family intact, in other words, if they were able to bring their disabled child with them. There is, therefore, a need for innovative, holistic models of respite services such as special resorts where families can bring their disabled child (and their well children) that are designed to provide restorative vacation time to families by providing care for the disabled child.

For those families who might not use other respite models, this type may break them into the idea of using respite services in a gentle way. Early intervention will reap the greatest benefits.

VARIABLES

A respite model that allows families to vacation as a unit experiencing restorative, relaxing and playful time together will strengthen families and their coping mechanisms. If families take advantage of respite care early in the disability, it will have beneficial effects on the family's long-term coping strategies and their utilization of other respite models. The informal networking of similarly challenged families (i.e., father to father, mother to mother, siblings to siblings) and socialization opportunities for the child with a disability would have great therapeutic effects for all family members.

ASSUMPTIONS

It is assumed that the families will answer the survey honestly. It is assumed that family vacation time is a wholesome and positive activity that families would like to enjoy together. It is assumed that siblings would benefit from time spent with their parents while they are free from the care of their disabled brother or sister (i.e., the disabled child would be taken care of by someone else at the resort). It is also assumed that siblings of disabled children, while playing together, will reap therapeutic benefits and that their relationships with their parents will also be reenforced by the leisure time together.

DEFINITION OF TERMS

The following definitions will apply to this discussion:

1. *Holistic:* "A holistic perspective of leisure is one that recognizes and integrates multiple factors affecting leisure behavior. Social, psychological, economic, cultural and personal and environmental variables are all thought to contribute to the leisure choices made by individuals and to the meanings that individuals attribute to leisure" (Howe-Murphy and Charboneau 1987).

2. *Disabled developmentally:* For the purposes of this study, "disabled" will include those children who chronically require partial to full assistance in activities of daily living.
3. *Families:* For the purposes of this study, "families" will include primary caregivers, the child with a disability and those they live with.
4. *Early intervention:* Services that target families as close to the diagnosis of the disability as possible so as to develop and maintain healthy patterns of coping.
5. *Family systems:* An approach to the delivery of services which identifies family needs, locates the informal and formal resources and support for meeting those needs, and helps to link families with the identified resources (Hobbs et al. 1984, in Dunst et al. 1988).
6. *Respite care:* A system of temporary supports for families and caregivers of developmentally disabled individuals, which provides the family and caregiver with relief from care provision (NICHEY 1989).

REVIEW OF THE LITERATURE

There is a social cost associated with the challenge of meeting the needs of the disabled. Caregivers who spend an average of 8.8 hours a day caregiving (Beecher 1988) experience social isolation and show a lack of participation in their community (Bader 1985; Cobb 1987; Sabbeth 1984). They experience financial difficulties and their health suffers (Holroyd and Guthrie 1979; Sabbeth 1984; Bader 1985). Because most caregivers in our society are women, this is primarily a women's health issue. Not only are our communities deprived of the participation of women who must spend the majority of their time as caregivers, but so is the work force as many of these women were forced to abandon educational and career goals due to the care demands of their children (Beecher 1988; Knoll and Bedford 1989; Holroyd and Guthrie 1979; Sabbeth 1984). Families experience increased stress and decreased functioning (Holroyd and Guthrie 1979) and there is an increased risk of neglect and abuse of the disabled child (Bader 1985; Subramanian 1985). All of the family systems are affected and thus the need for a holistic approach to services.

Caregivers, when surveyed, are primarily concerned with their child's welfare and secondly with relief for themselves. They are concerned with stress and finances as well as their own emotions and health. They would like to spend more time with their spouses and other children and have more opportunities for family interactions and mutual activities

(Beecher 1988; Cobb 1987; Knoll and Bedford 1989; Versluys 1986). Can respite care meet some of these needs and allay some of these costs, both social and financial?

Although there is not a great deal of research on the benefits of respite use, those studies that have been conducted demonstrate positive effects. Among caregivers there has been documentation of an increase in satisfaction with life, hopefulness about the future, ability to cope, improved attitude about the child and a decrease in aggregate maternal stress, pessimism and perception of the child's burden (Appolloni and Triest 1983; Rimmerman 1989; Cohen 1982; Marc and MacDonald 1988). Among families the benefits of respite have been proved to be an increase in family social functioning and a decrease in parental and family problems and family stress (Cohen and Warren 1984; Cohen 1982; CSR 1989; Marc and MacDonald 1988; Halpern 1985; Wikler and Hanusa, in Cohen and Warren 1984). For the disabled, respite has prevented their institutionalization (Cohen 1982; Cohen and Warren 1984; Joyce and Singer 1983; Pagel and Whitling, in Cohen and Warren 1984; CSR 1989) and their abuse (Subramanian 1985). These results would lead one to believe that there is no reason for not using respite care services, but the reality is that many families do not.

Those who do use respite seem to be the neediest. In studies comparing users to nonusers, users had less personal supports, were particularly needy, experienced extreme care demands, had more children and were more likely to be single-parent households (Beecher 1988; Cohen 1982; Robinson 1987; Marc and MacDonald 1988).

When given the free time, how do most people use it? The most common uses of respite care are for entertaining and socializing, leisure, self and family development, vacations, personal activities, rest and recuperation, and improving relationships with other family members (Beecher 1988; Cohen 1982; Cohen and Warren 1984; Halpern 1985; Aanes and Whitlock 1975; California Institute on Human Services, in Cohen and Warren 1984). This use of "free" time is surprising because with all the daily challenges these families are faced with, their main priority is recreation.

Most of those who do not take advantage of respite services are hesitant to leave their child (Beecher 1988; Cohen and Warren 1984; Devlin 1986; Green and Evans 1984; Halpern 1985; HSRI 1989). This hesitancy is attributed to worry, guilt, fear of being perceived as unloving or unable to cope, denial of their circumstances and concern about the possible inadequacy of respite workers (CSR 1989; Devlin 1986; Green and Evans 1984; Robinson 1987; Salisbury and Intagliata 1986; Edgar et al. 1988; Halpern 1982 and Hagen et al. 1980, in Cohen and Warren 1984;

HSRI 1989). Cost was cited in a few studies as a deterrent to use (Walker et al. 1988; CSR 1989). How can human service professionals address some of these concerns and coax nonusers into using the benefits cited earlier? The answer is in early intervention.

It has been shown that for families caring for a disabled member, stress-related problems increase over time and as the disability progresses (Holroyd and Guthrie 1979; Rimmerman 1989). A national survey of siblings found that the highest level of need for family support was when the disabled sibling was younger and school-aged (Itzkowitz 1990). According to Rimmerman and colleagues (1989), respite is of most benefit to mothers who have a high sense of self-esteem and who have young developmentally disabled children, and Joyce and Singer (1983) found that families whose children were recently disabled reported receiving more benefits from respite services than families whose children had been disabled for a longer period of time. One key finding of the Rimmerman (1989) study was that availability and accessibility bear no influence on respite use. Rather, all measures of respite utilization are related to self-esteem, family cohesion and adaptation. Thus, families need to experience respite before the long-term effects of caregiving demands compromise the characteristics that allow for the optimal use and benefit of the services—a chicken-and-egg dilemma of sorts, unless there is a choice of models that overcome the barriers to use that were cited earlier. Less threatening models, ones that for the purpose of family recreation and leisure provide an environment of therapeutic and restorative interactions for all family members early in their challenge, will have long-lasting, positive effects on coping resources and enhance use of other family support services and models of respite care.

When parents in various studies were asked how respite can better meet their needs, they asked for more respite time, more overnight respite, improved quality of workers, a higher ease of use, more respite in the form of day care and a continuum of services in every community with different models to match family needs (NICHEY 1989; Knoll and Bedford 1989; Beecher 1988; Cohen 1982; CSR 1989; Zirul et al. 1989). When asked how they might structure an ideal respite program, families identify a number of adjunctive services that they think might make respite more accessible and more useful to them. These services include:

1. Babysitting for siblings
2. Worker freedom to accompany families on outings to help care for the child
3. Brief respite relief periods for parents while the child is in the hospital

4. Before and after school care and summer day care
5. Parent support groups
6. Parent workshops on aspects of disabled child care (e.g. CPR)
7. Social events to bring families together
8. Discussion groups with parents and respite providers to encourage joint problem solving
9. A centralized respite referral agency or clearinghouse
10. Levels of care for children with special medical or behavioral problems
11. Same-day availability or emergency respite care

The parents felt that the inclusion of any of these services in a respite care program would increase its sensitivity and responsiveness to family needs (CSR 1989). Seven of these eleven services would be incorporated into a vacation resort model for these families (numbers 1, 2, 5, 6, 7, 8 and 10 above). There is much support in the literature from professionals and parents themselves for the need for, and positive benefits of, networking and informal associations among parents, siblings and children with disabilities. There is an increased understanding of the emotional ramifications of parenting a child with a disability such as feelings of guilt and anger or hesitancy to accept the child. For some fathers these informal opportunities are the only chance they have to discuss their feelings, especially with other fathers. There is support and comfort in knowing that others understand, that there is a referral to appropriate resources and an avoidance of unnecessary use of more costly alternatives such as seeking physician's advice or assistance (CSR 1989; Levy and Levy 1990; Perrin and Ireys 1984; Salisbury and Intagliata 1986; Versluys 1986; Zirul et al. 1989).

METHODOLOGY

The study was conducted using survey design. The population studied was made up of families who were challenged by the care of a child with a disability. The sampling frame was all those families in the New York City area who might attend a camp fair and the sample was those families who did attend the Camp Fair in New York City at The Jewish Guild for the Blind on Sunday, February 3, 1991 from 10:30 a.m. until 4:00 p.m., who consented to answer the survey. The Young Adult Institute allowed me enough space at their display table to hang a poster to attract parents and families and to have them sit and complete the survey. The poster read: "Do You Need a Vacation? Please Take a Few Minutes to Answer a Ten-Question Survey." There was no selection process on my part other than to invite those whose interest was sparked by the poster to sit for a few minutes and complete my survey. The families had the option of taking the survey and later mailing it to me or completing it there; all chose the latter. It became apparent that the opportunity to sit down was an incentive to filling out the survey. Twenty-six surveys were completed.

The instrument, the Family Vacation Survey, was designed to identify the vacation patterns and needs of families. Although not pretested, several revisions of the survey were made based on the recommendations of Dr. Judy S. Itzkowitz from the Sibling Information Network. I started by explaining the purpose of the survey and what I intended to do with the information obtained. I assured that confidentiality would be maintained and nowhere in the survey would personal information such as name, address or phone number be solicited.

The subjects were asked to complete the questions in order of their presentation as the design of the survey was such that later questions could bias responses to earlier ones. The earlier questions sought a current or baseline orientation toward the concept of a vacation and later questions sought responses to the proposed new model. I sought to ascertain whether, after having the new model concepts to consider as possibilities, attitudes toward vacations would be altered.

The survey consisted of 10 questions and an option to make any additional comments about vacation needs or patterns. Most questions were multiple choice, but there was also the option to write out an answer and most questions offered the option of circling more than one answer. The subjects were asked to take their time and dream a little about the possibilities presented.

The first two questions were supposed to determine the relationship of the person completing the survey to the disabled child and the nature of their family's makeup (i.e., number of siblings, parents, other adults and the age of the child with a disability). Questions 3 to 5 asked if a vacation was something these families wanted or something they were accustomed to taking. They were also asked when was the last time they took a vacation and if they had not taken one, what their main reasons were. Questions 6 and 7 were to determine what type of vacation a family would most likely choose: with or without the special child; with other similarly challenged families; with workshops for different family members, etc. Question 8 asked about the importance of a family vacation and was designed to validate the question—Is a family vacation something you would like to take? Question 9 asked for yearly household income and question 10 asked specifically about whether my proposed respite (family resort) model would be of interest to them.

RESULTS

The majority of respondents (73 percent) were women and the mothers of a child with a disability. The children with disabilities were for the most part 4 to 40 years old; 62 percent were between 4 and 10 years old, 15 percent were between 11 and 18, and 19 percent were over 18. A great majority (88 percent) of disabled children had one or two siblings; 70 percent lived with both parents and 26 percent lived with one parent. Their average household incomes were more or less equally divided between under $25,000, $26,000 to $46,000, $46,000 to 65,000 and $66,000 and above.

In testing my hypothesis (the major points of which are indicated by italics), *given the present selection of respite care services many families are not able to get that needed break in the form of a vacation.* In fact, 59 percent of those who answered my survey do not take vacations. Most of the respondents (61 percent) did not want to leave their child or felt that taking the child with them wouldn't seem like a vacation and 42 percent stated that finances were the major obstacle. Twenty-nine percent responded that they had never taken a vacation since starting their family and 24 percent said that they hadn't taken a vacation since the birth of their child with a disability. A small number (6 percent) said they regularly took vacations without their disabled child.

Families would take vacations if they could keep their family intact and have a break from the routines and demands of caring for the child with a disability and their able-bodied children. Responses show that there is a great desire to take a family vacation (85 percent) and if they could take their child and be relieved of the child's care, they would prefer that type of vacation. Four of the nine respondents who selected a vacation site specifically for families with a member with a disability also wanted to take their disabled child if specialized babysitting services were readily available at the vacation site. Of the remaining five there was an assumption that choice C included babysitting. Based on this assumption, 81 percent of the subjects preferred the proposed model. Even among the seven who responded that they would prefer to vacation without their disabled child (while the child is at camp or with a caretaker of their choice), three indicated that they would prefer to vacation as a whole family.

There is a need for innovative, holistic models of respite services such as special resorts designed to provide restorative vacation time to families challenged with the care of a disabled member. These models need to preserve the family unit as these families prefer to vacation with respite available at the vacation site. Family recreation in the form of a vacation was very or somewhat important for 96 percent of the respondents. Eighty-five percent indicated that they would prefer to vacation as a complete family, the same number who answered that a family vacation is something they would like to take.

Most of the respondents showed an interest in new models that provide organized recreational activities and workshops, particularly the opportunities for informal networking in a relaxed environment among similarly challenged families. Only three of the respondents indicated that they would prefer not to vacation with similarly challenged families and all of those who answered this way said they wanted to vacation with their disabled child if specialized babysitting services were readily available at the vacation site.

For those families who might not use other respite models this type may break them into the idea in a gentle way and promote healthier attitudes toward separation throughout the special child's life. Early intervention of these models will reap the greatest benefits in this regard. Of those respondents claiming that they would not leave the child for a week or have not vacationed since the birth of their child, 46 percent felt that family recreation in the form of a vacation was very important and would prefer to vacation as a complete family. Thirty-five percent of those who claimed that taking the child with them would not feel like a vacation opted for the on-site babysitting model.

Fathers' responses, although only 15 percent of the total, were tabulated to determine differences. In answer to the question, Is a family vacation something you would like to take? 50 percent of fathers said yes and 50 percent said maybe or would prefer a vacation without children. Interestingly, a full 100 percent said that they would prefer to vacation as a complete family versus 88 percent of the survey total. This supports the reasoning behind having the questions answered in order. In response to the question, How important is family recreation in the form of a vacation? 50 percent said "somewhat" versus 50 percent "very important." This differed from the survey total of 73 percent versus 23 percent. Fathers were less likely to opt for leaving the child behind, 75 percent said they would not leave the disabled child for a week (versus 23 percent of the survey total). Seventy-five percent of fathers opted for professionally conducted recreational group activities.

Especially noteworthy was the fact that, at the beginning of the survey, 42 percent of respondents claimed that their reason for not taking a family vacation was financial and at the end of the survey none of these respondents chose the statement: Would be nice but could not afford a vacation. Of these 42 percent, 18 percent had household incomes over $66,000, 27 percent had incomes between $46,000 and $65,000, 9 percent between $26,000 and $45,000 and 36 percent between zero and $25,000. Perhaps they wouldn't, as opposed to couldn't, pay for the present models available.

The final question of the survey allowed for any additional comments about vacation needs or patterns. The responses were:

- It is important to have both options; family vacation is important but so is time for both parents and child independently.
- This type of service should be offered at time-sharing condominium retreats.
- The best vacation I ever had was when the ski instructor kept the child busy most of the day. I was nearby and knew he was safe and I really had a vacation.
- I would prefer a regular vacation like any other family, such as to DisneyWorld.
- I would like to know more about dealing with this issue.
- Our ideal vacation would be to take our children and have the option of leaving our autistic son with caregivers while we explored areas and still have him near for the activities we can do with him.
- I feel family vacation should include all members. Fortunately my son does not have a great many medical needs; our biggest problem is affording everything.
- A vacation is like recharging a battery.
- The major restriction was the severity of the condition and the discomfort in leaving.

SUMMARY AND CONCLUSION

The findings of this study determine the need for early intervention models of respite care that keep the family intact for the purpose of family recreation and leisure. Although the sample was small, it showed surprisingly consistent responses supporting the hypothesis. These families were at a camp fair and were already motivated to seek a separate model of respite in the form of camp. These were families who had sufficiently overcome the barriers of leaving their special child to consider the possibility of camp. Even among families who would send their child to camp there was much support for taking their disabled child with them on a family vacation if the appropriate models were available. Perhaps they would still send their child to camp as another form of respite for them. Ideally there should be as many alternative and varied forms of respite as there are needs.

What about the families who were not at the camp fair, who will not consider leaving their child in the care of others at all, much less for an extended period of time? It would seem likely that their support for a family resort model of respite services would be stronger even than those at the fair. There must be a large number of families that never get the needed break from the challenge of caregiving, a large number of families who do not recreate together, a large number of siblings who never share relaxed time with their parents, a large number of couples who never have playful, leisure time together—all because a child with special needs is born. There is a need to develop innovative, family-centered models of respite to lessen this impact and eliminate the negative associations.

I do not believe that the survey results would have been much different in the general population of families with 4 to 10 year olds except that perhaps they will not have foregone a vacation. However, the general population has options like Club Med, which accommodates families and keeps the children entertained all day. Human service professionals should recognize that these families need all the services other families need, but that they have some special needs. Day care, school holiday and summer programs allowing parents to have full-time jobs and vacation resorts that provide on-site respite or babysitting are among the needs of all families wishing to participate fully in society. These families do not start out any different than others. They become isolated and stressed and dysfunctional over time as they meet barriers to a "normal" life. Early intervention models that reassure them that they can want and have what everyone else has and wants will alter the psychological course of adjustment to their family member with a disability toward a healthier acceptance and level of functioning.

I propose an inn type of resort for these families, a place where they can be together with other families in an environment that is relaxing, strengthening and therapeutic in a casual, intimate sense. This inn would be staffed by summer interns and instructors in the human service fields as well as competent respite workers. There would be a very rich environment for interventions and studies for and of parent groups, sibling groups and groups of disabled children. It could be an institute in an inn setting, providing a vacation to families and a rich environment for researchers. I would like to see control group studies done with such a model to measure many things, including levels of stress before and after intervention for families coming with their special child and those leaving their child in the care of others. Much knowledge could be gained in the design of services for families challenged by the care of a disabled member.

I have dealt specifically with new models of respite for families newly challenged with the care of a disabled child. However, caregivers of disabled family members are in the category of adult children of disabled parents as well and the geriatric literature is swelling with articles on respite. How do these families recreate? Perhaps some research could be done to determine the prevalence of the inability to leave their parent in this population of caregivers.

More research should be done on non-users of respite care so that their needs can be more appropriately met. More longitudinal studies need to be done to find out the long-term effects of early intervention on the prominent complaints of these families (e.g., isolation, stress, the stigma siblings deal with and the general level of family dysfunction). Attention needs to be paid to those completed studies that tell human service professionals that parents want versatility in service models. Parents want input in the design of services. An early emotional bolstering of these families will produce long-term benefits for the disabled children, their families, the communities they live in and our society in general. Failure to intervene early can only promote the use of more costly alternatives for all of these systems.

REFERENCES

Ahmann, E. An annotated bibliography on respite care for children and families. *Children's Health Care* 14(3):183-186, 1986.

Ames, L. A rest for parents of the disabled. *The New York Times,* January 27, 1991, p. WC 33.

Apolloni, A.H. and G. Triest. Respite services in California: status and recommendations for improvement. *Mental Retardation* 21:240-243, 1983.

Bader, J. Respite care: temporary relief for caregivers. *Women & Health* 10(2-3):39-52, 1985.

Baker, J. and R. Michael. A windfall for disabled kids. *Newsweek* 110(9):72, 1987.

Beecher, R. Respite Care's Influence on Mothers of Children with Developmental Disabilities. Ph.D. dissertation, Brigham Young University, 1988 (*Dissert. Abstr. Int.* 49[5]:A1091).

Cobb, P.S. Creating a respite care program. *Exceptional Parent* 17(5):31-33, 36-37, 1987.

Cohen, S. Supporting families through respite care. *Rehab. Lit.* 43(1-2):7-11, 1982.

Cohen, S. and R. Warren. *Respite Care: Principles, Programs and Policies.* Austin, TX: Pro-Ed Publishers, 1984.

CSR Incorporated and U.S. Department of Education. *Respite Care is for Families: A Guide to Program Development.* Washington, DC, 1989.

DeSalvatore, G. Therapeutic recreators as family therapists: working with families on a children's psychiatric unit. *Therapeutic Recreation J.* 6:23-28, 1989.

Devlin, R. Respite care: holiday home. *Community Outlook* 9:5-6,11, 1986.

Dunst, C., C. Trivette and A. Deal. *Enabling and Empowering Families: Principles and Guidelines for Practice.* Cambridge, MA: Brookline Books, 1988.

Edgar, E., P. Reid and C. Pious. Special sitters: youth as respite care providers. *Mental Retardation* 26(1):33-37, 1988.

Green, J.M. and R.K. Evans. Honeylands' role in the pre-school years: II. Patterns of use and III Factors inhibiting use. *Child* 10:81-98, 1984.

Halpern, P. Respite care and family functioning in families with retarded children. *Health and Social Work* 10(2):138-150, 1985.

Holroyd, J. and D. Guthrie. Stress in families of children with neuromuscular disease. *J. Clin. Psychol.* 35(4):734-739, 1979.

Howe-Murphy, R. and B. Charboneau. *Therapeutic Recreation Intervention: An Ecological Perspective.* Englewood Cliffs, NJ: Prentice-Hall, 1987.

Human Services Research Institute. *Support for Families of People with a Disability: Bibliography and Resource Guide.* Cambridge, MA: HSRI, 1990.

Human Services Research Institute. *Family Support Services in the United States: An End of Decade Status Report.* Cambridge, MA: HSRI, 1990.

Human Services Research Institute. *Becoming Informed Consumers: A National Survey of Parents' Experience with Respite Services.* Cambridge, MA: HSRI, 1989.

Itzkowitz, J. Siblings' perceptions of their needs for programs, services, and support: a national study. *Sibling Information Network Newsletter* 7(1), 1990.

Joyce, K. and M. Singer. Respite care services: an evaluation of the perceptions of parents and workers. *Rehab. Lit* 44(9):270-274, 1983.

Killian, K. Respite care and the therapeutic recreator. *Therapeutic Recreation J.* 18(1):27-30, 1984.

Knoll, J. and S. Bedford. Respite services: a national survey of parents' experience. *Exceptional Parent* 19(7):34-37, 1989.

Levy, J. Families with disturbed children: why don't they recreate? *Am. Therapeutic Recreation Assoc. Newsletter* 1:15, 1985.

Levy, J.M. and P.H. Levy. Impact of Adolescent Disability Upon the Family. In Emanuel Chigier, ed., *Youth and Disability.* London: Freund Publishing House, 1990.

Luginbill, M. and A. Spiegler. A community-based program for children with special needs. *Children Today* 22:5-9, 1989.

Marc, D.L. and L. MacDonald. Respite care: who uses it? *Mental Retardation* 26(2):93-96, 1988.

McNulty, B. and L. Goodwin. Who should be served, where and why: local special education administrators' views. *Topics in Early Childhood Special Ed.* 8(3):51-60, 1988.

Monroe, J. Family leisure programming. *Therapeutic Recreation J.* 4:45-51, 1987.

National Information Center for Children and Youth with Handicaps (NICHEY). Respite care: a gift of time. *NICHEY News Digest* 12, 1989.

Newacheck, P., P. Budetti and P. McManus. Trends in childhood disability. *Am. J. Public Health* 74(3):232-236, 1984.

Perrin, J. and H. Ireys. The organization of services for chronically ill children and their families. *Pediatric Clin. North Am.* 31(1):235-257, 1984.

Ptacek, L., P. Sommers and J. Graves. Respite care for families of children with severe handicaps: an evaluation study of parent satisfaction. *J. Community Psychol.* 10(3):222-227, 1982.

Rimmerman, A. Provision of respite care for children with developmental disabilities: changes in maternal coping and stress over time. *Mental Retardation* 27(2):99-103, 1989.

Rimmerman, A., R, Kramer, L. Levy and P.H. Levy. Who benefits most from respite care? *Int. J. Rehab. Res.* 12(1):41-47, 1989.

Robinson, C. Key issues for social workers placing children for family based respite care. *Br. J. Social Work* 17:257-284, 1987.

Sabbeth, B. Understanding the impact of chronic childhood illness on families. *Pediatric Clin. North Am.* 31(1):47-57, 1984.

Salisbury, C. and J.Intagliata. *Respite Care: Support for Persons with Developmental Disabilities and Their Families.* Baltimore: Paul H. Brooks Publishing, 1986.

Subramanian, K. Reducing child abuse through respite center intervention. *Child Welfare* 64(5):501-509, 1985.

U.S. Department of Education. *Summary of Data on Handicapped Children and Youth.* Washington, DC: Human Services Research Institute, National Institute on Handicapped Research, 1985.

U.S. General Accounting Office. *Respite Care: An Overview of Federal, Selected State, and Private Programs.* Washington, DC: GAO, 1990.

U.S. Senate. *A Compilation of Federal Laws for Disabled Children, Youth and Adults.* Washington, DC: Subcommittee on the Handicapped, Committee on Labor and Human Resources, 1985.

Upshur, C. Developing respite care: a support service for families with disabled members. *Family Relations* 32:13-20, 1983.

Versluys, H. Thuishulpcentrale: a Dutch model for practical family assistance. *Rehab. Lit* 47(3-4):50-58, 1986.

Walker, D., J. Palfrey, et al. Use and sources of payment for health and community services for children with impaired mobility. *Public Health Rep.* 103(4):411-421, 1988.

Zirul, D., A. Lieberman and C. Rapp. Respite care for the chronically mentally ill: focus for the 1990s. *Community Mental Health J.* 25(3):171-184, 1989.

21

Respite Care in
the Nursing Home:
Predictors of Length of Stay*

Jeanne A. Teresi, PhD and Audrey S. Weiner, MPH

Generically, respite care is defined as socially sanctioned temporary care of the frail elderly and disabled to permit family caregivers to relinquish their duties and responsibilities (and also their stress) for limited periods of time (Miller et al. 1986; Miller and Goldman 1989). Respite services may include "planned, intermittent, short-term" acute care (Hasselkus and Brown 1983), day care and in-home care for community-resident impaired elderly. Hegeman's (1989) study of 75 existing respite programs throughout the United States found that 15 percent of the respite providers offered in-home respite exclusively, and another 6 percent offered in-home respite in combination with one or more respite models, most typically a nursing home/in-home combination. Community-based respite programs, including adult day care programs and freestanding respite facilities, represented 41 percent of all survey respondents. Within the institutional milieu, geriatric respite care is being provided by skilled nursing facilities (40 percent), intermediate care facilities (31 percent), adult homes (17 percent) and senior housing (4 percent). Some investigators (Yatzkin 1989) have argued that long-term institutionalization

* The authors acknowledge the support of the Columbia University Alzheimer's Disease Research Center—Research, Training and Information Transfer Core Project and the Center for Geriatrics and Gerontology in the preparation of this chapter.

should be considered as the ultimate form of respite care. However, for the purpose of this discussion, respite care is defined as continuous day care to the impaired elderly who are residents of the community. Respite care is assumed to be restorative in terms of the mental and physical health of caregivers and an implicit goal is the reduction of long-term institutional care days.

As with many concepts and programs in the field of geriatrics, there is a precedent for their development to be found in models applied to other disabled populations and age groups. There is a fairly extensive body of literature on respite care programs for impaired children and adults; most focus on developmentally disabled children; however, there are many evaluations of respite programs for individuals with such illnesses as epilepsy, cerebral palsy, autism (Cohen and Warren 1985) and schizophrenia (Grad and Sainsbury 1963). Many of these programs date to the early and mid 1960s. Review of the respite research in other areas is of interest in that programmatic elements and evaluation outcomes of elderly respite programs parallel those of the earlier programs designed for other age groups and disabled populations.

The conclusions drawn from evaluations of over 20 such respite programs servicing non-elderly clients are that (a) the respite programs are frequently used by families with small extended informal support systems; (b) the services are used for the more severely impaired individuals; (c) in-home respite is preferred over "out-of-home" services; (d) families express great satisfaction with respite; however, (e) respite care is only effective if a sufficient amount of respite time is provided by the program. (See Cohen and Warren [1985] for a more detailed review.) Major reasons for termination of respite or for agency refusal to continue clients on respite include severe behavioral disorders and major medical conditions. Claims are made that respite care enhances family interactions and reduces the risk of long-term institutional care. The high economic cost of institutionalization, the belief that community living best supports the quality of life of older adults and the fact that the family is a major health care provider have motivated health planners and providers to explore respite as a programmatic option (Hasselkus and Brown 1983). However, results regarding the impact of respite care are inconclusive.

During the last several years there have been many evaluations of respite services to the elderly; however, very few were based on experimental designs or panel studies. Much evidence regarding respite care is anecdotal or correlational; however, based on these studies it has been concluded that families report better patient-family interactions (McIntyre and Brink 1983; Sands and Suzuki 1983); improved health

(Scharlach and Frenzel 1986) and a high degree of satisfaction with services (Lawton, Brody and Saperstein 1989; Scharlach and Frenzel 1986; Weissert 1989). More prevalent reasons for use of respite services include emotional rest (Scharlach and Frenzel 1986); physical rest (Hasselkus and Brown 1983; Scharlach and Frenzel 1986); catching up with chores or needed medical treatments (Miller and Goldman 1989) and recreational or social activities. Caserta and co-workers (1987) have ranked the reasons caregivers give for not using services: perceived lack of immediate need; reluctance to leave their patient with strangers; feeling the relative was too behaviorally impaired; and financial reasons. Lawton and associates (1989) reported that the reasons for nonuse of respite in their experimentally designed intervention study were so diverse that no specific categorizations could be made.

Caserta's group (1987) reported that caregivers waited as long as possible to seek respite services. This is similar to the findings of Montgomery and co-workers (1989), who found that 40 percent of their sample were deceased or in nursing homes within 1 year of the initiation of respite care, indicating that caregivers were seeking help only in the endstage of illness. Lawton's group (1989) reported that caregivers wait until "late in the caregiving process or when crises occurred to seek help." The Caserta team (1987) also noted that those caregivers who were not ready for services (43 percent) had significantly lower measured burden and higher social support and their relatives were less functionally demented.

Results are equivocal regarding reduction of long-term institutional care as a result of respite. For example, Scharlach and Frenzel (1986) reported that while 33 percent of caregivers felt that institutional placement was less likely than it would have been without respite, 30 percent felt that institutionalization was more likely because clients already had experienced the institutional setting. Caregivers found institutional placement beneficial and less threatening than they had anticipated. Moreover, the experience made caregivers more aware of their caregiving burden.

The few available experimental, quasi-experimental and longitudinal studies show that while client satisfaction with respite services is high, there is limited "hard" evidence of their efficacy. Burdz and co-workers (1988) applied a three-way mixed-model multivariate analysis of variance (MANOVA) to compare the outcome of respite intervention provided to demented and nondemented elderly. A total of 55 caregivers were interviewed 2 to 7 days prior to respite care provision and again 14 to 21 days after respite termination, using a burden inventory and memory and behavior checklist. Of this sample, 35 families received respite placement and the remaining 20 formed the waiting list group. The results did not support the hypothesis that respite relocation would be relatively more detrimental to dementia patients; the problem scores of all respite group patients decreased in relation to the comparison group. The respite group caregivers reported lower levels of burden than did the caregivers on the waiting list, but this difference was not significant.

Montgomery's group (1989) conducted a longitudinal evaluation over 3 occasions (baseline, 12 and 20 months) of the impact of five intervention packages on objective and subjective caregiver burden and nursing home placement. The sample consisted of 541 volunteers who were randomly assigned to one of the five groups or to a comparison group. The sample included spouses, children and other caregivers and their care recipient. The intervention group packages included various combinations of support seminars, support groups, respite and family consultation. The major finding of the study, using repeated ANOVA measures, was a reduction in subjective burden among spouses in the respite group. Results regarding rates of nursing home placement were equivocal, given the relatively small prevalence of nursing home placement and cell sizes for some analyses.

Lawton's team (1989) conducted a study of 317 experimental group subjects who received one or more of the following paid respite services: in-home care, day care and short-term institutional care and 315 control subjects who were not offered respite services. The respondents were followed up 12 months after initial interview. Respondents were first recruited into a caregiving research project; a criterion for acceptance into the program was cognitive impairment as measured by a score of 7 or more on the Kahn-Goldfarb Mental Status Examination and a physician diagnosis of mental impairment. Respondents were then randomly assigned to experimental or control groups. Survival and multiple regression analysis showed no significant differences between experimental and control groups in terms of time, measures of caregiver health and well-being, after controlling for initial levels of each. The results of a survival analysis examining community tenure for the impaired elderly indicated that the experimental group spent 22 days longer in the community than did the control group, a statistically significant, but small effect. The Lawton group concluded that respite care is a modestly effective intervention in terms of most outcome variables; however, most respite recipients endorse it. Weissert and co-workers (1989), based on their earlier research and on results from a nationally representative sample of 60 adult day care centers, similarly concluded:

though previous research has shown that neither costs nor participant outcomes appear to be favorably altered by day care, and the current analysis shows that—regardless of model—most participants are at low risk of nursing home residency, participants and their caregivers are overwhelmingly satisfied with the care they receive (p.649).

Callahan (1989) argues that endorsement and satisfaction are not enough and that a persuasive argument for respite care can only be made in terms of "hard" outcomes such as reduction in costs of care. Capitman (1989), in response to Weissert's analyses, commented that the researchers must determine which sets of services are best for particular sets of caregivers and older clients, as well as under what circumstances and for how long.

Caregivers frequently identify respite as a needed service; for example, Caserta's group (1987) identified respite care as accounting for 71.3 percent of the reported service needs of a nationwide sample of 597 primary caregivers. Although caregivers identify the need, the service is frequently not used or is underused. A major finding of Montgomery and colleagues (1989) was the difficulty in recruiting subjects and getting them to avail themselves of services. Most (91 percent) of one treatment group used family consultation (home visits), but many did not use any of the other services. The Lawton team (1989) reported that caregivers "needed considerable time, education, and encouragement to begin to understand and use respite."

Given the substantial difference between actual use and expressions of need, it is not surprising that acute and long-term care facilities are wary of providing services; only 30 percent of the members of the American Association of Homes for the Aging, the national umbrella for nonprofit long-term care providers, offer residential respite programs.

This chapter will examine predictors of length of stay among users of adult day health care services, providing an overview of clients and their decision making regarding the use of respite.

DESCRIPTION OF PROGRAM

The day care program is under the auspices of the Hebrew Home for the Aged at Riverdale (HHAR), an 1100-bed nonprofit, nonsectarian long-term care facility located in the Bronx, New York. The Samuels Adult Day Services Center (SADSC) opened in December 1986, consistent with regulations of the New York State Department of Health for a medical-social model program. The purpose of this adult day health services program is to:

1. Restore or maintain the client's optimal physical, emotional and cognitive functioning.
2. Provide respite and support to caregivers.
3. Enable an individual to remain in the community as long as possible.

These major goals are accomplished within a center that:

1. Includes structured cognitive and social stimulation and recreation.
2. Coordinates health care needs, specifically providing specialty medical services (i.e., psychiatry, neurology and cardiology), core medical services as defined by the regulations (i.e. dental, podiatric and ophthalmologic services) as well as physical therapy, occupational therapy, speech therapy and audiology.
3. Links this program with other community services to avoid duplication and ensure consistency of clinical and supportive approaches.
4. Provides a respite to families, as well as education and support to both families and paid caregivers.
5. When appropriate and necessary, eases the transition to nursing home care.

This particular center has focused on meeting the needs of those with moderate to severe dementia in the community. Based on the premise that homogeneous client placement according to functional level is optimal to meet the program goals, three program tracks have been developed:

1. The *Special Care* program for individuals with a diagnosis of dementia who are at the moderate to severe stage of the disease, characterized by disorientation to time and place, and often person; deterioration of short-term memory, verbal abilities and social skills; incontinence; wandering; and occasional agitation.
2. The *Integrated* or *Mainstream* track, which includes those individuals at the mild to moderate stages of dementia, with psychiatric and neurologic disorders, as well as those who are physically frail but cognitively intact.
3. A *"Bridging the Gap"* program option for individuals with moderate dementia who have retained socially acceptable behaviors and can participate and acclimate to the activities and structure of tracks 1 and 2 above.

Transfer between tracks occurs as the client's condition changes. Presently, individuals attend the Special Care (SC) track 3 days a week: Monday, Tuesday and Thursday. Wednesday and Friday are program days for the Integrated track. Clients in the "Bridging the Gap" (BG) track may attend anywhere from 2 to 5 days depending upon their needs.

Transportation by contract ambulette is provided for 97 percent of the clients and is available for those who live within a 30-minute radius of the Center. Clients are picked up between 7 and 9 in the morning; the program day ends at 3 in the afternoon. However, from the perspective of providing respite for family members or the opportunity to continue to work, transportation can be arranged so that clients are picked up as early as 7 a.m. and returned home as late as 4:45 in the afternoon.

The program has an approved capacity of 40 persons per day and an average enrollment of 88 clients. The program is staffed by a full-time coordinator, a registered nurse, a social worker, a recreation worker, a secretary, four full-time program/nurses' aides, a part-time recreation aide and a music specialist. Medical, occupational and physical therapy, speech/audiology and dietitian services are provided by the nursing home by contract.

DESCRIPTION OF THE MEASURES

The respite care admission process begins with a telephone call for information and is followed by a nursing, psychosocial and financial assessment at the Center, using the Respite Assessment Inventory (RAI). Medical information, including a medical order to participate in the program, is required prior to admission. Family members are asked the reasons for admission to the Center as an open-ended question on the initial application. The 28-item Blessed Mental Status Test (Blessed, Tomlinson and Roth 1968) is used to measure memory and orientation. Information on basic ADLs and mobility is obtained using the Patient Review Instrument (PRI).

Sixteen case-mix index categories are designated, with "PA" (Physical A) denoting the highest level of ADL function, and hence the least level of services required in the areas of eating, mobility, transfer and toileting. A PA category means that the individual scored from 0 to 4 on the four ADLs, where each ADL score ranges from 0 to 4 or 5. Length of stay (LOS) was measured by converting the interval between date of admission and date of discharge into days of program stay.

DESCRIPTION OF THE SAMPLE

The sample is composed of 248 Day Center participants from December 1986 through December 1989 attending three program tracks. The average Day Center participant's age is 80.89 years. Average attendance is 2.6 days per week. Forty-four percent of the cohort are married and living with their spouse but 80 percent of all males are married. Only 20.6 percent of the participants (nearly all in the Integrated track) are able to live alone. In total, 40 percent of all clients are male. In the Special Care track the percentages of men and women are almost equal; in the Integrated track 64 percent are female.

The average length of stay in the program ranges from 264 days in the SC track to 313 days in the Integrated track. Individuals in the BG track are in the program longest—390 days, reflecting admission at earlier stages of the dementing process.

One-fourth of the participants are supported by Medicaid. Of those paying privately (6.9 percent) the majority are charged by means of a sliding fee scale. The sliding fee scale, available because of private foundation support, makes the Center accessible to working- and middle-class families in New York City.

Not surprisingly, given the auspices of the Center and its location in a middle-class white community, 89.5 percent of the clients are Caucasian, 7.7 percent are Black, 2 percent are Hispanic, 64 percent are Jewish, 22.7 percent are Catholic and 8.5 percent are Protestant.

There is significant diversity in client education and occupation. For example, approximately equal numbers of clients (one-fourth) have less than a ninth grade education or have attended college. Similarly, client occupations show variety with the majority of women having been housewives or held clerical positions. Of those remaining, 13.1 percent were skilled workers, 10.7 percent semi-skilled and 11.9 percent minor professionals.

Dementia (SDAT, MID and mixed) is the most prevalent of all diseases, affecting 83 percent of the Special Care track, 71 percent of the Bridging the Gap track and 16 percent of the Integrated track participants. Average Blessed Mental Status scores by track are: Integrated (6.90), BG (14.9) and Special Care (20.93). The Bridging the Gap track participants do, in fact, score between those in the Special Care and Integrated tracks. Individuals with psychiatric or neurologic impairments are included; more (26.8 percent) of the Integrated track than the SC track participants (5.1 percent) have suffered strokes, and are thus more impaired in ambulation. More (13.4 percent) of the Integrated track than the SC track participants (4.7 percent) have been diagnosed as depressed, a frequent concomitant of stroke. Typical of the age of the population, cardiovascular disease, arthritis, diabetes and Parkinson's disease also affect significant numbers of participants.

A "rest" or "relief" was identified by caregivers as the reason for seeking day care respite in 58.5 percent of the cases (43.8 percent in the Integrated and 75.3 percent in the Special Care track). While dementia is the "reason" given in 13.6 percent of the applications, the impact of a dementing illness and other chronic conditions is reflected in phrases such as "to maintain independence" (43.8 percent in the Integrated and 16.8 percent in the SC track).

CONCEPTUAL MODEL AND TESTS OF BIVARIATE HYPOTHESES

Bivariate and multivariate analyses were conducted, examining correlates and predictors of length of stay for the 248 day care participants. Analyses were performed using a conceptual model based on results of previous research, on our clinical experience and observations regarding respite services and on a service utilization model proposed by Anderson and Newman (1973).

A conceptual model was employed for the study of the research hypotheses. It was assumed that predisposing, enabling and need factors relate to length of stay. While the conceptual model posits both direct and indirect effects (predisposing and need factors through enabling factors), the current analyses examine only direct effects. The model posits that service use is dependent on an individual's predisposition (demographic characteristics and beliefs), how enabled the individual is to obtain services and the degree of need (illness level). A number of factors have been hypothesized as impacting on length of stay (LOS) in the day center. These relationships are examined first in bivariate fashion and then in terms of the unique saliency of each factor in predicting LOS in the multivariate context. Multivariate relationships are examined for both the Special Care and the Integrated track samples. It is important to examine each separately because one of the criticisms of respite day care programs is that they have not properly assessed and targeted consumers so that unique programs can be provided, based on level of cognitive function.

There are marked differences between the Special Care and Integrated track samples in the targeted direction. The following are some significant associations of SC membership with other variables. SC clients are more demented (r=.67); less depressed (r=−.14); have fewer medical problems (r=−.16) such as stroke, diabetes and arthritis; and are more impaired in eating (r=.17), but less impaired in ambulation (r=−.13). The SC clients tend to be males; married and living with spouse (r=.22);

non-Jewish (r=−.21); and referred so that caregivers could have some respite (r=.31) rather than in an attempt to maintain independence in the community (r=−.29). SC and Integrated participants do not differ significantly in major PRI categories.

Hypotheses

1. *Dementia severity will be related to shorter length of stay. This relationship will be stronger in the Special Care sample.*

The use of respite services at earlier stages in the caregiving or dementia cycle may enable respite to have more of a preventive quality (Lawton, Brody and Saperstein 1989; Miller and Goldman 1989) and hence be more effective. Once the client is more demented, institutional placement is more likely.

This hypothesis was supported at the bivariate level; those with high Blessed scores stayed in day care for significantly shorter periods of time (r=−.15; p<.05). This negative association obtained for all samples. Dementia was not a significant variable in the multiple regression analyses.

2. *Higher ADL function will be related to increased length of stay. This relationship will be stronger in the SC sample.*

The NCOA summary of *Adult Day Care in America* (Behren 1986) identifies incontinence and degree of mobility impairment (i.e., wheelchair-bound or cannot transfer without assistance) as reasons for *exclusion* from admission to day centers across the country. A related finding that "24-hour care was too difficult" was offered as the reason for institutionalization by 72 percent of caregivers of demented relatives in a study by Chenoweth and Spencer (1986). This phrase was considered to include all aspects of ADLs. While the Samuels Adult Day Services Center does *not* limit participation by these criteria, it is anticipated that the potential to remain in the community is greater if the related physical and emotional strain on the caregiver is minimized.

This hypothesis was supported; the PA PRI categorization, which is the case-mix index category reflecting highest independence and ADL function, was highly predictive of length of stay for both SC (r=.36) and Integrated (r=.32) samples. This variable was uniquely salient in predicting LOS in regression analyses across samples. Of interest is that mobility impairment was related to *longer* LOS in the total and Integrated samples, but not in the SC sample. Mobility was a significant predictor in the regression analysis for the total sample.

3. *The spouse as the primary caregiver, especially if female, will be related to decreased length of stay. The relationship between spouse caregivers and length of stay will be stronger in the SC sample.*

Lund, Pett and Caserta (1987) found that spouses of individuals with dementia perceive the likelihood of institutionalization to be significantly lower than adult children and friends who assume the caregiver role. Caregiver responsibilities are viewed, in this context, as fundamental aspects of the marital relationship. It is predicted that spouses will be more likely to remain in day care if their only alternative is long-term institutional care. On the other hand if the spouse caregivers come to the program at advanced stages of caregiving, the client may be closer to institutionalization. The day care clients of spouse caregivers are significantly more likely to be males, younger than other clients (r=–.21), demented (r=.26), parkinsonian (r=.13) and in the SC track (r=.22). The spouse caregivers overwhelmingly come to day care for respite (r=.57) rather than for reasons such as "maintaining the client's independence in the community" (r=–.30). Within the Special Care track of the Center, 50 percent of the clients are male; the majority are cared for by their spouses. Most female clients are cared for by children, who are likely to be caring for families of their own and thus are experiencing role overload (Colerick and George 1986).

This hypothesis was supported; clients of spouse caregivers are significantly less likely to remain in the program (r=–.13); there is a tendency for the relationship to be stronger in the SC than in the Integrated track.

4. *Participants living with paid, nonfamily members, in contrast to children, will be related to increased length of stay and to less frequent discharge to nursing home.*

It is hypothesized that being cared for by paid, nonfamily members would result in a reduction of the number of hours and intensity of direct caregiving by children. Opting for nursing home care, in lieu of a community service option, would not be anticipated to be as likely. This hypothesis was not confirmed; paid, nonfamily caregiving was not related (r=.01) to LOS or to discharge to nursing home (r=.02). This finding is similar to that of the Channeling evaluation (Mathematica Policy Research 1986) and the Kibbutz study (Holmes et al. 1989) where it was found that substitutability of formal for informal supports is not a deterrent to institutionalization.

5. *Medicaid as a source of payment will be related to increased length of stay.*

The average cost of day care (even with a sliding fee scale) at the Center is $62.52 per day including transportation. This is a considerable expense for middle- and working-class families, and may be a barrier to respite service use (Duke Family Support 1990). Medical model day care is a Medicaid-reimbursable service in New York State. As a result of the 1990 changes in Medicaid regulations regarding transfer of assets and spousal refusal to pay, the percentage of Medicaid clients increased in the Center from 23 to 43 percent between 1987 and 1989. It is hypothesized that the availability of Medicaid assistance will result in finance being a less salient predictor of program attrition.

This hypothesis was not confirmed for the total or Integrated sample, and for the SC sample the opposite relationship was observed. Private pay (rather than Medicaid) reimbursement was significantly related to length of stay at both the zero order level (r=.17) and in the multivariate context. Special Care sample participants with Medicaid reimbursement stayed in the program an average of 203.11 days as contrasted with non-Medicaid recipients (mean LOS=285.03 days). Private pay SC track clients tend to be males (r=.39), tend to have had strokes, and tend to be discharged from the program to nursing homes (r=.17) or to hospital (r=.15). Two-thirds of the private pay SC participants are spouses as contrasted with one-fourth of the Medicaid SC participants.

6. *Family identification of "respite" as a reason for program use will be related to decreased length of stay.*

It is hypothesized that by the time the family can identify a *need* for respite services, the caregiver has experienced some dimension of burden and the disease processes which have prompted admission to the Center have progressed significantly. This hypothesis was not confirmed; the correlation of respite as a reason for application with LOS ranged from 0 to −.04 across samples.

7. *Families' articulation of "remaining in the community" and "maintaining independence" as goals of admission are related to increased length of stay. It is hypothesized that this relationship will be stronger in the Integrated track.*

The families' approach to a program goal based on the client's well-being suggests a client who is at a higher level of function (physically or cognitively), a family member for whom the relief from burden is not yet a priority (i.e., respite) and a clear direction in desired outcome.

This hypothesis was borne out at the bivariate level; the relationship for maintaining independence as a reason for Center use and length of stay correlated .30 for the total sample. Counter to prediction, the relationship was stronger for the SC sample (r=.40) than for the Integrated sample (r=.20).

8. *Physicians as a referral source will be related to increased length of stay.*

Referral from a physician may give the earlier use of respite services professional sanction. Gonyea and co-workers (1988) suggest that family caregivers regard the use of formal respite care as valid when their emotional or physical health is seriously jeopardized; nonetheless caregivers are less likely to seek such supports for emotional, spiritual or physical renewal. Practitioners, especially physicians, who include respite as part of the entire treatment plan, are more apt to make this intervention in a preventive context. The combination of sanction, feeling less abandoned and more capable as a result of concrete physician suggestion (Chenoweth and Spencer 1986) will be related to increased length of stay.

This hypothesis was not confirmed; in fact physician referral was related to *shorter* length of stay for the total and for the integrated samples, and was significant in the multivariate analysis. This relationship is puzzling in that physician referral was not significantly related to dementia, ADL impairment or many other variables.

9. *Special Care track status will be related to shorter length of stay.*

Special care track patients have more severe dementia. Mace and Rabins (1984) found high rates of discharge from adult day centers to nursing homes or as a result of death. This may indicate that these individuals are suffering from a chronic deteriorating disease such that their length of stay in day care is limited. In their national survey of 980 day centers, the rate of discharge in centers with a higher percentage of dementia clients supported the impression that the centers are caring for a sicker cohort. These "centers" are analogous to the Special Care track in the Samuels Adult Day Services program. The discharge rate to nursing homes is 17.8 percent in the SC track and 11.6 percent in the Integrated track.

There was modest support for this hypothesis; SC status was related negatively to length of stay (r=−.11, p<.05), while integrated status was not. The mean length of stay for SC clients is 263.60 days, while the average LOS for the integrated sample is 313.40.

MULTIVARIATE ANALYSIS

Hierarchical multiple regression analyses were performed using the same model, entering the same variables, in the same order for each subsample (SC and Integrated track). The rationale for the order of entry was that it was desirable to first determine the extent to which individual client need characteristics alone accounted for variance in LOS. Enabling factors (such as Medicaid payment status) and predisposing demographic variables, referral sources and presenting problems or beliefs were entered, followed by reasons for discharge.

Those who stayed in day care longer were significantly more likely to be depressed, less ADL-impaired, but more impaired in mobility; they tended to have fewer sources of referral to the program, were referred from sources other than a physician and caregivers of these participants reported more reasons for referral. Those who stayed for shorter periods of time tended to leave because their caregivers were no longer interested; they were too ill to attend; or were placed in nursing homes or hospitals.

Nearly half (42 percent) of the variance in days of attendance was accounted for by the variables in the model: the majority (21 percent) by ADL/ambulation, 10 percent by reasons for discharge, 7 percent by presenting problems and 5 percent by referral sources. Need factors accounted for 25 percent of variance and enabling for none. Predisposing variables accounted for 12 percent of the variance: 1 percent for demographics, 5 percent for referral sources and 6 percent for beliefs (reasons for seeking respite).

Within the SC sample, significant predictors of LOS in the multivariate context were being less ADL-impaired, having fewer sources of referral and being private pay. Shorter length of stay is predicted by leaving for reasons of lack of interest, nursing home placement and relocation. Selection of day care with a goal of maintaining independence was almost significant. Altogether 45 percent of the variance was explained: 14 percent by ADL impairment, 10 percent by referral sources, 9 percent by choosing respite to maintain independence, 8 percent by discharge reasons, and 4 percent by private pay as opposed to Medicaid status.

The results for the Integrated track subsample show that depression and mobility disorder are associated with longer stay. Older participants stayed longer. ADL impairment and physician referral are associated with shorter stay. Those with more presenting reasons for seeking respite services stay longer, as do those with better attendance during the first month of day care.

About half (51 percent) of the variance in length of stay was accounted for, with mobility accounting for 23 percent, ADL function for 7 percent, depression for 6 percent, presenting reasons for 5 percent. Reasons for discharge accounted for an additional 10 percent of the variance.

A comparison of the SC and the Integrated track indicates that the major differences in the prediction of length of stay are to be found in the relative importance of mobility. Ambulation difficulty is a much more salient predictor of longer stay for the Integrated sample. Additionally, the number of presenting problems, depression and attendance during the first month are uniquely salient. For the SC sample, better ADL performance and fewer sources of referral are important in predicting longer stay. Private pay clients and those who seek day care to maintain independence are likely to stay longer. These latter variables were not uniquely salient for the Integrated sample.

In terms of the Anderson-Newman model, there is a difference between tracks in the amount of variance explained by each category of variable. Among the Integrated track participants, 39 percent of the variance in length of stay was explained by need factors, while predisposing factors were less important: 2 percent, demographics; 9 percent, referral sources and 5 percent, beliefs. Enabling factors accounted for no variance. On the other hand, for the special care track, the most important factors were not need (19 percent), but predisposing conditions (25 percent), including demographics (3 percent), referral sources (12 percent) and beliefs that respite care would enhance independence and provide rest (10 percent). Enabling factors accounted for 4 percent of the variance.

DISCUSSION

The univariate analyses show that similar to the findings of other researchers (Lawton et al. 1989; Scharlach and Frenzel 1986, Weissert 1989), respite and day care users express great satisfaction with services. Those family members seeking residential and day care respite services tend to come to the program because they are caring for relatives with dementia. Those in the Special Care track, where participants have greater cognitive dysfunction, tend to choose day care for reasons of rest rather than to maintain independence. Maintaining independence is a more prevalent reason for Integrated track members. However, within the SC track, choosing respite to maintain independence is a uniquely salient predictor of longer stay.

The multivariate analyses show that need factors such as basic ADLs and particularly mobility impairment, along with discharge due to illness, play a greater role in predicting length of stay for the Integrated rather than the SC sample, with those who stay longer having more impairment in ambulation (frequently associated with strokes), but less impairment in basic ADLs such as eating and toileting. For SC track clients, predisposing factors, particularly caregiver beliefs that coming to the program will maintain client independence (in contrast with coming for respite)

is a more salient predictor of LOS than for the Integrated track participants. Perhaps those caregivers who come for this reason are either not
yet "at their wit's end" as caregivers or are more motivated to maintain
their relative in the community. The former reason is supported to some
extent in that the spouses in the SC track are caring for more dysfunctional relatives, with more basic ADL impairment than the daughters
and other caregivers in the track. Spouses tend not to come to day care
to "maintain independence." Thus the relationship between LOS and
choosing respite to maintain independence may be moderated by level
of impairment.

In summary, the results show that for these samples, dementia is
associated with fewer medical problems, more impairment in basic ADLs
(e.g., eating and toileting), but less impairment in mobility. SC track
clients have more severe dementia and stay less time in the day care
program. Integrated track clients (who on the average are less cognitively
impaired and less mobile) stay longer. In general, across tracks, those
who are less impaired in basic ADLs remain in the programs longer.

Separate examination by the authors of the reasons for not using
respite services (among those who applied but did not enroll) indicates
that the major reason for not pursuing the service is rejection by family
or client either because they don't like to be with other "sick" people or
because they don't feel quite ready yet. This latter finding may correspond
with the findings of others (Caserta et al. 1987; Lawton et al. 1989;
Montgomery et al. 1989) that respite care is used late in the caregiving
cycle. In the current study, about two-fifths (36.6 percent in the Integrated
track and 41.1 percent in the SC track) were discharged from the program
because they were too ill to attend, were placed in a hospital or nursing
home, or died.

Research in this area suggests that the goal of respite as a preventive
rather than a crisis service has yet to be achieved. Additional public
relations addressing the nature of these services, targeted outreach to
physicians and community agencies, and better linkage with the
Alzheimer's Association information and referral groups remain as objectives.

Additional research is needed to better target respite resources
according to level of client and caregiver need. An examination of the
process of caregiver decision-making regarding use or non-use of services
would facilitate a better understanding of those who are summarily
labeled "resistant" or "uninterested."

REFERENCES

Anderson, R. and J.F. Newman. Societal and individual determinants of medical care utilization in the United States. *Milbank Memorial Fund Q.* 51:95-124, 1973.

Behren, R.V. *Adult Day Care in America: Summary of a National Survey.* Washington, DC: National Council on Aging and National Institute on Adult Day Care, 1986.

Blessed, G., B. Tomlinson and M. Roth. The association between quantitative measures of dementia and senile changes in the cerebral grey matter of elderly subjects. *Br. J. Psychiatry* 114:797-811, 1968.

Burdz, M.P., W.O. Eaton and J.B. Bond, Jr. Effect of respite care on dementia and non-dementia patients and their caregivers. *Psychology and Aging* 3(1):38-42, 1988.

Callahan, J.J., Jr. Play it again Sam—there is no impact. *Gerontologist* 29(1):5-6, 1989.

Capitman, J.A. Day care programs and research challenges. *Gerontologist* 29(5):584-585, 1989.

Caserta, M., D.A. Lund, S.D. Wright and D.E. Redburn. Caregivers to dementia patients: the utilization of community services. *Gerontologist* 27(2):209-214, 1987.

Chenoweth, B. and B. Spencer. Dementia: the experience of family caregivers. *Gerontologist* 26(3):267-272, 1986.

Cohen, S. and R. Warren. *Respite Care: Principles, Programs and Policies.* Austin TX: Pro-Ed, 1985.

Colerick, E.J. and L.K. George. Predictors of institutionalization among caregivers of patients with Alzheimer's disease. *J. Am. Geriatrics Soc.* 34:493-498, 1986.

Deimling, G.T. Respite use and caregiver well-being in families caring for stable and declining Alzheimer's disease patients. Benjamin Rose Institute, 1990.

Grad, J. and P. Sainsbury. Mental illness and the family. *The Lancet,* March 1963, pp. 544-547.

Gonyea, J.G., G.B. Seltzer, C. Gerstein and M. Young. Acceptance of hospital-based respite by families and elders. *Health and Social Work* 13(3):201-208, 1988.

Hasselkus, B.R., and M. Brown. Respite care for community elderly. *Am. J. Occup. Ther.* 37(2):83-88, 1983.

Holmes, D., J. Teresi, M. Holmes, S. Bergman, Y. King and N. Bentur. Informal vs. formal supports for impaired elderly people: determinants of choice on Israeli kibbutzim. *Gerontologist* 29:195-202, 1989.

Lawton, M.P., E. Brody and A. Saperstein. Respite care for Alzheimer's families: research findings and their relevance to providers. *Am. J. Alzheimer's Care Related Disorders Res.* November/December 1989, pp. 31-38.

Lund, D.A., M.A. Pett and M.S. Caserta. Institutionalizing dementia victims: some caregiver's considerations. *J. Gerontol. Social Work* 11(1/2):119-135, 1987.

Mace, N.L. and P.V. Rabins. Day care and dementia. *Generations* 9(2):41-44, 1984.

Mathematica Policy Research. Channeling effects on informal care. Washington, DC: U.S. Department of Health and Human Services, 1986.

McIntyre, E. and T.L. Brink. Families over-predict improvement of elders in day care. *Clin. Gerontol.* 1(3):94-95, 1983.

Miller, D. and L. Goldman. Perceptions of caregivers about special respite services for the elderly. *Gerontologist* 29(3):408-410, 1989.

Miller, D., N. Gulle and F. McCue. The realities of respite for families, clients, and sponsors. *Gerontologist* 26(5):467-470, 1986.

Montgomery, R.J.V. and E.F. Borgatta. The effects of alternative support strategies on family caregiving. *Gerontologist* 29:457-464, 1989.

Sands, D. and T. Suzuki. Adult day care for Alzheimer's patients and their families. *Gerontologist* 23(1):21-23, 1983.

Scharlach, A. and C. Frenzel. An evaluation of institution-based respite care. *Gerontologist* 26(1):77-81, 1986.

Weissert, W.G. Models of adult day care: findings from a national survey. *Gerontologist* 29(4):640-649, 1989.

Yatzkin, E. Correlates of Demoralization in a Cohort of Spousal Caregivers of Alzheimer's Victims. Unpublished doctoral dissertation, New York University, 1989.

22

Adult Day Care:
A Comparison of Users
and Nonusers*

Audrey S. Weiner, MPH and Jeanne Teresi, PhD

Within the past decade, adult day care has established itself as a key option in the continuum of care for the chronically ill and disabled in the United States (O'Brien 1982; Weissert et al. 1990). The national increase in the number of adult day centers during the past decade parallels both the growth of the dependent elderly population that requires supportive services and the improved funding prospects under the Medicaid Home and Community-Based Care Act of 1981 (Title XIX, Medicaid Section 1915c; Weissert et al. 1990). In 1989, the National Institute on Adult Day Centers identified approximately 2100 adult day care programs across the country.

Lindeman and co-workers (1991) suggest that day care is an important option for caregivers who often become physically and mentally exhausted by having to provide constant care to an elderly or disabled relative. In that context, it offers support consistent with the classic definition of respite care as "... socially sanctioned temporary care of the frail elderly and disabled to permit family caregivers to relinquish their duties, stress and responsibilities for time-limited periods" (Miller et al. 1986; Miller and Goldman 1989).

* The authors acknowledge the support of the Columbia University Alzheimer's Disease Research Center—Research, Training and Information Transfer Core Project and the Center for Geriatrics and Gerontology in the preparation of this chapter

In fact, the National Institute on Adult Day Care (1990) identifies the provision of respite to the caregiver as an appropriate goal of adult day care programs. Relatedly, the New York State Department of Health's client assessment form for adult day health programs includes "support for the informal caregiver" as a legitimate reason for program use.

Despite the recognition of the value of adult day care programs from the perspective of respite as well as other services, family members are not "flocking to program doors" (Lindeman et al. 1991). Although community-based needs assessments document strong interest in adult day care programs (Caserta et al. 1987; OTA 1987; Weiner, Reingold and Holmes 1990), there is a disparity between perceived need and actual usage. This differential between a positive needs assessment and actual usage can be termed "negative demand." In other words, the consumer needs the service but will go to great lengths to avoid its use (Lindeman et al. 1991).

Documentation of the underuse of adult day centers is provided by Weissert and associates (1990) in their in-depth national study of 60 day care centers; they note the median occupancy of all-day centers to be 80 percent. Centers that operate under the auspices of either nursing homes or rehabilitation hospitals operated at 67 percent of occupancy and those under the auspices of general hospitals, social service or housing agencies operated at 80 percent of capacity. In his 1983 report on adult day services in Massachusetts, Palmer found a similar pattern of below-capacity operation that was attributed to variable absenteeism. That report noted that even though day centers operate below capacity, programs had to "staff up" to capacity on a regular basis. Operating at below capacity is a concern from three perspectives:

1. Are programs meeting clients' and families' needs?
2. What is the cost in terms of quality and diversity of programs and lost income of operating below capacity?
3. What is the cost to the program and those individuals who apply to adult day centers and do not enroll?

Kirwin (1988) indicates the need for research to predict patterns of resistance to using available formal services—i.e., is there a difference between the clients who will use adult day care and those who will not when there is equal accessibility?

The purpose of this chapter is to describe and contrast, using the experiences of one center, a group of 669 individuals who have applied to an adult day services center during a 4-year time span, 37 percent of whom have enrolled in the program; 63 percent have chosen not to enroll. The multivariate data analysis will focus on identifying the determinants of program use among 155 individuals who were assessed during an in-person interview; 109 later enrolled in the program while 47 did not.

DESCRIPTION OF THE PROGRAM

The Samuels Adult Day Services Center (SADSC) is a program of the Hebrew Home for the Aged at Riverdale (HHAR), a nonprofit and nonsectarian long-term care facility in the Bronx, New York. The program, organized under the umbrella of the Brookdale Center for Community Care, was developed following a 1-year planning study conducted to determine the needs of individuals with dementing illnesses and their families.

While the study indicated that a full continuum of care was needed in this community, adult day health care was, in fact, identified as a high priority (Weiner, Reingold and Holmes 1989). The Samuels Adult Day Services Center opened in December 1986, consistent with the regulations of the New York State Department of Health for a medical model program. The Center has focused on meeting the needs of those with moderate to severe dementia in a format discrete from those who are physically frail. Based on the premise that homogeneous client placement according to functional level is optimal to meet program goals and client needs, three program tracks (discussed in the last chapter of this book) have been developed: the Special Care (SC) program for individuals with a diagnosis of dementia who are at the moderate to severe stages of the disease; the Integrated track, which includes those individuals at the mild to moderate stages of dementia; and a "Bridging the Gap" (BG) program option for individuals with moderate dementia who have retained socially acceptable behaviors and can participate and acclimate to the activities and structures of the Special Care and Integrated tracks.

Social skills, behavioral function, verbal competence and cognitive status as determined by a comprehensive assessment, including the Blessed Mental Status Test (Blessed, Tomlinson and Roth 1968), as well as family and physician input determine placement by track.

As of July 30, 1991 there were 92 clients on the roster and an average daily census of 38.2. There was also a waiting list for services. A certificate of need application has been filed for expansion of the program's size from 40 visits or clients a day to 75 visits a day to meet the expressed needs of the client cohort for more days per week and longer hours per day, as well as to respond to the waiting list.

In 1990, the number of visits to the Adult Day Services Center was

9412, in contrast to 8819 in 1989. During 1990 there were 233 requests for applications to the program and 25 percent of these applicants were admitted.

DESCRIPTION OF THE SAMPLE

The samples used for this study include:

1. The 248 Samuels Day Services Center participants from December 1986 through December 1989. This group includes a subsample of 109 individuals who were initially assessed using the same format and data collection instruments as subgroup b below.
2. The 421 individuals who applied to the Samuels Adult Day Services Center and chose *not* to enroll during approximately the same time period.

The group of 421 was examined as two subgroups:

a. The 374 individuals about whom demographic information was obtained via a telephone screen or brief application.
b. The 47 individuals who were assessed at the Center by a clinical member of the staff for whom information about diagnosis, reasons for referral and referral sources was also available.

DEMOGRAPHIC OVERVIEW

A comparison between the 248 program participants and program applicants on key demographic variables shows the following information. The average age of the day center participant was 80.89 years, in comparison to the average age of the applicants which was 80.71 years and the average age of individuals who are assessed at the Center which was 80.34 years. Sixty percent of the participants and 62 percent of the applicants were female. The spouse was the primary caregiver for 44 percent of the participants and 29 percent of the applicants. One-fourth of the participants were supported by Medicaid; of the applicants, 14.7 percent were on Medicaid.

REASONS FOR NONUSE

Reasons for nonuse of services suggested in the literature include: financial concerns; guilt and anxiety over sharing caregiver responsibilities (Caserta et al. 1987; Duke Family Support Center 1990); lack of adequate or accessible care; and failure to properly target clients (Deimling 1992). In this context we examined reasons for nonuse of the adult day services center.

During 1990, only 25 percent of those callers who requested information about the day center actually became enrolled in the program. Data for all 421 persons contacting the day center from December 1986 to February 1991 were examined to determine their reported reason for nonuse.

Retrospective examination of the reasons for nonuse of day care indicated that the major reasons that *families* rejected the Center (occurring for 24.4 percent of the cases) included "family just seeking information for later"; "not ready at this time"; "other clients in the program are too ill"; and "family members are resistant." The *client* rejected the Center in 15.7 percent of the cases. Other reasons for nonadmission together with the number of those giving them, included:

Illness, hospitalization or death	42 (10.0%)
Nursing home placement	28 (06.7%)
Financial reasons	23 (05.5%)
Other day program was more suitable	16 (03.8%)
Moved out of area	10 (02.4%)

Admission to the Center typically occurs within a process that begins with a request for information and includes a brief application; on-site nursing, psychosocial and financial evaluation; community physician's medical orders for admission and the actual admission. For the 669 individuals who initiated the process by a telephone call (or in rare instances a drop-in visit) from 1986 to 1990, the following steps in the process were completed (these steps are typically but not necessarily sequential):

Application requested and mailed	640 (95.6%)
Application returned	328 (49.0%)
Assessment appointment scheduled	378 (56.5%)
On-site assessment completed	295 (44.1%)
Primary community physician completes history/physical and orders for admission to the Center	281 (42.0%)
Admitted	248 (37.0%)

CONCEPTUAL MODEL AND TESTS OF BIVARIATE HYPOTHESES

A series of hypotheses was developed and examined in an effort to describe the differences between the applicant and client groups. The analysis builds on Anderson and Newman's 1973 model of predicting service use based upon the complex relationships of the predisposing, enabling and need factors. Predisposing factors are those individual characteristics that affect the recognition of illness. Need factors (both actual and perceived) are those variables that affect the decision to take action, and the enabling factors affect the actual start and use of a service. Within this data set, the specific variables are organized as follows:

Predisposing Factors	*Need Factors*	*Enabling Factors*
Age	Actual need (diagnosis)	Financial status (i.e. Medicaid eligibility)
Gender		
Religion		
Caregiver/patient relationship	Perceived need (reasons for referral)	
Referral sources		

Hypotheses

The analyses for hypotheses 1 and 2 below are based on the larger samples for whom sociodemographic data were available (n = 248 participants and 421 applicants).

1. *If the primary caregiver is the spouse, it is more likely that the client will be admitted to the Samuels Adult Day Services Center.*

Lund, Pett and Caserta (1987) found that spouses of individuals with dementia perceive the likelihood of institutionalization to be significantly lower than adult children and friends who assume the caregiver role. Caregiver responsibilities are viewed, in this context, as fundamental aspects of the marital relationship. It is predicted that spouses will much more likely choose day care services if the alternative is long-term institutional care. This hypothesis was supported.

2. *Medicaid as a source of payment will be related to admission to the program.*

The average cost of the day center (even with a sliding fee scale) is $68.60 per day including transportation. This is a considerable expense for middle- and working-class families and may be a barrier to service use (Duke Family Support Center 1990). If an applicant already has Medicaid as a source of payment for this program, it is not likely that concerns regarding the financial implications of the program will be a barrier to accessing services. This hypothesis was supported.

3. *Neither age nor gender (of the caregiver and/or the patient) will be related to admission to the Samuels Adult Day Services Center.*

The client's age has not been noted as having a relationship to burden (Zarit, Reever and Bach-Peterson 1980; George and Gwyther 1986; Pratt, Wright and Schmall 1987; Novak and Guest 1989; Cohen and Eisedorfer 1988), although the model of stress of Pearlin and co-workers (1990) suggested that background and context, including socioeconomic characteristics, do impact on service use. However, in Miller's (1990) semi-structured interview with 15 caregivers of cognitively impaired spouses, it was noted that both husbands and wives agreed to assume authority over their memory-impaired spouse. While husbands took charge without questioning their ability to do so, wives were less comfortable and confident. However, problem-solving techniques were used by caregivers of both genders and use of services is one problem-solving technique.

This hypothesis was partially supported; that is, age was not related to service use. However, that the potential client was female was related to increased likelihood of admission.

4. *Family identification of "respite" as a reason for program use will be related to admission to the Day Center.*

It is hypothesized that by the time the family can identify a need for respite services, the caregiver will have experienced some dimension of burden and, in that context, is willing to yield some of their caregiving responsibility. Pearlin's group (1990) provides a model for understanding caregiver stress in which one outcome, in this case the "yielding of role," is in fact related to primary stressors, secondary role strains (e.g., family conflict or constriction of social life) and intrapsychic strain. This hypothesis was supported.

5. *Of the total pool of individuals who call for information about the Center, those with dementia will be more likely to be admitted to the Center.*

It is hypothesized that such families are less likely to be "simply" seeking information as time demands of caregiving require more outcome-oriented activities. This hypothesis was not supported. One potential explanation is that it is related symptomology and disruptive or asocial behaviors of the dementia rather than its presence that would impact on service-use decisions (Pearlin et al. 1990; Wilder, Teresi and Bennett 1983). Such specific information is not available for these samples.

6. *Of the pool of applicants to the Center, those with depression will be more likely to be admitted to the Center.*

The authors' own analysis of SADSC clients indicated that depression was very positively associated with longer length of stay in the program ($r = .16$; $p < .05$). The caregiver's desire to respond to the relative's depression in a positive way is similarly hypothesized to be an enabling factor in completing the application process. This hypothesis was not supported.

7. *The greater the number of reasons for application, the greater the likelihood of admission to the Center.*

Adult day programs have traditionally publicized respite as a program goal and valid reason for use. Recently, however, Lindeman and co-workers (1991) suggested that marketing efforts for day centers focus on client as well as caregiver needs, and in that manner includes socialization and maintenance of independence. When the needs of both parties in the caregiver-client dyad can be met, it is hypothesized that admission to the center is more likely. This hypothesis was supported.

MULTIVARIATE ANALYSES

Logistic regression analysis was performed to determine the risk factors for participation vs. nonparticipation in the day care program. It was found that those who participated were significantly more likely to have chosen day care to foster independence. The older client was more likely to be female, to be Jewish and to be referred by a family or friend. Participants were less likely to have been referred by a physician or by HHAR staff; those with Parkinson's disease were significantly less likely to become participants; however, those with stroke were significantly more likely to enroll in the day care program. Variables that were significant correlates of participation in the bivariate analyses, but no longer significant in the multivariate context, included referral because of cognitive function or for socialization or respite.

This variable set is highly predictive of participation; using these variables, it is possible to correctly classify 96.8 percent of all individuals in terms of whether or not they participate. By far the most powerful variables are the reasons for entering this respite program; those caregivers who have more overall reasons for selecting this service option and those who want to enroll their relatives to maintain independence are far more likely to have relatives who actually participate in the day care program.

Examination of the Anderson-Newman model of service utilization for this sample shows the following: actual need variables (diagnosed medical conditions) accounted for 6.3 percent of the variance; perceived need characteristics (reasons for referral) account for 60.4 percent of the variance and increase the predictive ability (correct classification rate) by 21.1 percent. Enabling characteristics (Medicaid eligibility) add nothing to the ability to classify individuals as participants or non-participants. Predisposing characteristics account for 4.0 percent of the variance (demographics variables 1.9 percent, referral sources 2 percent and informal support: spouse 1 percent), and increase the correct classifications by only 5.1 percent. Thus, perceived need is the most important set of variables in terms of prediction of program participation.

SUMMARY

The data from the Samuels Adult Day Services Center indicate that during a 4-year time period, 37 percent of all callers requesting information actually enrolled themselves or their family members in the Center. Given that knowledge of the Center is not a barrier to service use for this population, differentiating service users from those who chose *not* to use the Center was the goal.

Of all callers, 44 percent are assessed at the Center, with 84 percent of all clients who are evaluated on-site actually enrolling. The loss of interest or follow-through is actually between initial contact and any one of the possible next steps (i.e., return of the application, scheduling of the assessment or completion of the assessment).

Consistent with Kirwin's (1988) recommendation to differentiate users from nonusers of service, bivariate and multivariate analysis was performed. Bivariate and multivariate analysis indicated that admission to the Center was more likely if:

- The primary caregiver was the spouse.
- The client was female.
- The caregiver was referred to the program by family or friends rather than by a physician.
- The client and/or family member identified a greater number of reasons for program use; particularly maintaining independence and respite from caregiving.
- The client suffered a stroke.
- The client did not have Parkinson's disease.

Multivariate analysis emphasized the role of perceived need characteristics or reasons for referral and indicated that 60.4 percent of the variance was explained by this variable set.

PROGRAM IMPLICATIONS

While adult day care, as a service modality, has been in existence for more than 21 years, its reality as a perceived resource by caregivers lags behind. Marketing and public relations for many centers has emphasized caregiver respite as a benefit of participation, even though the Center's program goals include maintenance of independence, maintenance in the community and socialization.

Given the indication in this data set that the caregivers believe that "maintenance of independence" is a legitimate reason for admission and as such is much more predictive of admission than a respite goal, programs should integrate the variety of service goals not only into promotional materials, but also program realities. In addition, it is recommended that if initial contact to the Center is made by telephone:

1. A knowledgeable staff member should obtain and convey information about the Center during the contact.
2. The information conveyed should include the multiplicity of possible program goals.
3. Calls followed up by clinical staff members should emphasize program opportunities for clients and caregivers.

This research focuses on a sample from one adult day health program affiliated with a nursing home. Based upon the research of Weissert and co-workers (1990), which shows significant differences among adult day care populations by auspices, additional research should focus on participation in different types of day care programs. This research should include interviews with caregivers regarding their reasons for program use and nonuse, the results of which would be of great benefit to practitioners and program advocates.

REFERENCES

Anderson, R. and J. Newman. Societal and individual determinants of medical care utilization in the United States. *Milbank Memorial Fund Q.* 51:95-124, 1973.
Blessed, G., B. Tomlinson and M. Roth. The association between quantitative measures of dementia and senile changes in the cerebral grey matter of elderly subjects. *Br. J. Psychiatry* 114:797-811, 1968.

Caserta, M.S., D.A. Lund, S.D. Wright and D.E. Redburn. Caregivers to dementia patients: the utilization of community services. *Gerontologist* 27:209-214, 1987.

Chenoweth, B. and B. Spencer. Dementia: the experience of family caregivers. *Gerontologist* 26(3):267-272, 1986.

Cohen, D. and C. Eisdorfer. Depression in family members caring for a relative with Alzheimer's disease. *J. Am. Geriatrics Soc.* 36:885-889, 1988.

Deimling, G.T. Respite use and caregiver well-being in families caring for stable and declining Alzheimer's disease patients. Unpublished manuscript, Benjamin Rose Institute, 1990.

Duke Family Support Center. *Overcoming Barriers to Appropriate Service Use: Effective Individualized Strategies for Alzheimer's Care.* Durham, NC: Duke Family Support Center, 1990.

George, L.K. and L.P. Gwyther. Caregiver well-being: a multidimensional examination of family caregivers of demented adults. *Gerontologist* 26:263-269, 1986.

Gonyea, J.G., G.B. Seltzer, C. Gerstein and M. Young. Acceptance of hospital-based respite by families and elders. *Health and Social Work* 13(3):201-208, 1988.

Jakobovitz, I. Ethical guidelines for an aging Jewish world. *J. Aging and Judaism* 2(3):145-157, 1988.

Kirwin, P.M. Correlates of service utilization among adult day care clients. *Home Health Care Services Quarterly* 9(1):103-115, 1988.

Lindeman, D.A., N.H. Corby, R. Downing and B. Sanborn. *Alzheimer's Day Care: A Basic Guide.* New York: Hemisphere, 1991.

Lund, D.A., M.A. Pett and M.S. Caserta. Institutionalizing dementia victims: Some caregiver considerations. *J. Gerontol. Social Work* 11(1/2):119-135, 1987.

Miller, B. and A. Montgomery. Family caregivers and limitations in social activities. *Research on Aging* 12(1):72-93, 1990.

Miller, D. and L. Goldman. Perceptions of caregivers about special respite services for the elderly. *Gerontologist* 29(3):408-410, 1989.

Miller, D., N. Gulle and F. McCue. The realities of respite for families, clients, and sponsors. *Gerontologist* 26(5):467-470, 1986.

National Institute on Adult Day Care. *Standards and Guidelines for Adult Day Care.* Washington, DC: National Council on Aging, 1990.

Novak, M. and C. Guest. Caregiver response to Alzheimer's disease. *Int. J. Aging and Human Dev.* 28(1):67-79, 1989.

O'Brien, C.L. *Adult Day Care: A Practical Guide.* Monterey, CA: Wadsworth, 1982.

Office of Technology Assessment, U.S. Congress. *Losing a Million Minds.* Washington, DC: U.S. Government Printing Office, 1987.

Palmer, H.C. Adult Day Care. In R.J. Vogel and H.C. Palmer, eds., *Long-Term Care: Perspectives from Research and Demonstration.* Rockville, MD: Aspen, 1983.

Pearlin, L.I., J.T. Mullan, S.J. Semple and M.M. Skaff. Caregiving and the stress process: An overview of concepts and their measures. *Gerontologist* 30(5):583-591, 1990.

Pratt, C., S. Wright and V. Schmall. Burden, coping and health status: Issues in the measurement of burden. *J. Gerontol. Social Work* 37:697-705, 1987.

Weiner, A.S., J. Reingold and D. Holmes. Planning to meet the needs of individuals with Alzheimer's disease: A case study. *Am. J. Alzheimer's Care Related Disorders Res.* 4(4):37-44, 1989.

Weissert, W.G., J.M. Elston, E.J. Bolda, W.N. Zelman, E. Mutran and A.B. Mangum. *Adult Day Care: Findings From a National Survey.* Baltimore: The Johns Hopkins University Press, 1990.

Wilder, D., J. Teresi and R. Bennett. Family burden and dementing illness. In R. Mayeau and W. Rosen, eds., *Recent Advances in Dementia.* New York: Raven Press, 1983.

Zarit, S.H., K.E. Reever and J. Bach-Peterson. Relatives of the impaired elderly: correlates of feelings of burden. *Gerontologist* 20:649-654, 1980.

23

Evidence of Goal Achievement: Evaluating Respite Programs

David E. Wilder, PhD

Among the problems that have accompanied development of respite services is a lack of clear definition of purpose or goals. There is no general consensus on the goals and objectives for respite care or on how and even whether these goals should be evaluated. For example, Callahan (1989) has argued that the overwhelming evidence is that respite services have failed to meet their stated goals of improving caregiver well-being and reducing institutionalization, that "the usefulness of a service should be measured against some criterion," and that there may even be social class and racial biases operating as reflected by patterns of usage and opportunity costs. In contrast, Lawton, Brody and Saperstein (1989) have argued that the relief and satisfaction that caregivers report are evidence enough that respite is intrinsically good; and they raise the question of whether respite services even need to be justified on the basis of their improving caregiver well-being or reducing the costs of care.

There is also a lack of agreement and uniformity as to what respite services are or should be. In our society, establishing programs with the intention of improving the quality of the lives of others must be done within the context of accountability, cost containment, third-party reimbursement, participant's rights, and numerous other legal and institutional constraints, with seemingly infinite varieties of state and local variations. It is tempting to argue that under such varying conditions, it is not possible to develop any viable system of respite services, much less gather credible evidence as to whether goals have been achieved. With these types of complexities and the relative infancy of the respite movement, it is not surprising that evidence of goal achievement is incomplete and uneven. But this incompleteness and unevenness may nevertheless provide sufficient opportunity to identify important gaps in our knowledge and suggest some of the types of research that would help to fill these gaps.

While conceived and developed in response to important and seemingly obvious social needs, respite services have often had difficulty getting started. It has not been clear from the outset what services should be provided, who should provide them, where they should take place, and how they can be funded. Sometimes even when funding has been forthcoming, space occupied, staffing and programs put in place, very few clients have shown up for the programs. Moreover, even well-established and pioneering respite programs may close down after many years of "successful" operation because they are not economically viable. In effect, the operation was successful, but the program died.

As policymakers and program planners have become more aware of the many problems they face in getting respite programs started and in keeping them going, some proponents have placed less emphasis on broad-based social and economic outcome goals, such as prevention of nursing home placements and cost containment, and more emphasis on humane goals, such as improving the quality of life of elderly persons with dementia and other chronic conditions and their caregivers. In addition, as program planners and evaluators have gained more experience with the realities of Alzheimer's disease and of the altered and stressful life circumstances it produces, more modest instrumental goals and objectives have been given attention, such as how to better match programs to clients' needs.

Given the lack of consensus about scope and purposes and the wide variety of existing respite forms and situations, it may be useful to review some of the important components of respite care for Alzheimer's disease in order to provide a better conceptual framework for evaluating respite programs and for clarifying the discussion of evidence of goal attainment.

The general definition of respite care is one of "temporary substitute care" that is provided for chronically, usually cognitively impaired persons who live in the community with the expectation that the usual caregivers will continue to provide care. It is not always clear from this definition whether some programs and services not usually considered to be respite, and which might have quite different stated goals or might better accomplish the goals set for respite care, should be included or excluded. For example, the word "temporary" would seem to exclude providing home health aides five afternoons a week for any extended period of time. Yet this type of home care might improve caregivers' quality of life and enable them to maintain care at home more effectively than would providing a "substitute" caregiver one or two afternoons a week. This problem occurs whether applying the usual definition of respite care to community-based or to institutional respite programs. The types of community and institutionally based respite care most frequently offered and evaluated are typically used so sporadically and for such short periods of time that it does not seem realistic to expect them to produce significant long-term or lasting effects. When respite care programs include only infrequent and very time-limited interventions, it makes sense to set more modest short-term goals and to reserve more substantial and long-term outcomes for more substantial interventions. This would help to avoid having to promote and justify many excellent respite programs on the basis of goals they probably cannot achieve.

It is often unclear where respite program boundaries reside and what should be included or excluded from the program, and this may also make evidence of goal attainment more difficult to obtain and evaluate. The simplest and sometimes most economical respite programs provide substitute care only, with the implicit assumption that this enables caregivers to do what they need or want to do during the periods of respite. In addition, many respite programs provide informational activities, case management and support groups for caregivers, and frequently this is done during the designated respite period. Medical model day care programs may also provide physical therapy, speech therapy, health assessment and other health-related activities. It is not always obvious whether or not these activities should be considered part of the respite program, and if they are part of the program, whether they contribute in any way to respite outcome goals.

At first glance the clients targeted by respite programs would appear to be a relatively unambiguous group. For example, we know from many studies that the majority of persons with dementia reside in the community and that they are cared for by family members who experience considerable stress over the period when they are responsible for providing care. It follows that respite care programs should target these caregivers and provide them with much-needed relief. However, sometimes very few caregivers utilize the programs designed for them. This has led to considerable soul-searching and examination of client needs and of reasons why targeted clients fail to make use of respite programs. In addition, although respite is by definition intended to benefit caregivers, programs such as day care are also frequently justified on the basis of their targeting and benefiting dementia patients as well as their caregivers. Social model programs provide socialization, reality orientation and a variety of other scheduled activities in group settings with the expectation that these will help their elderly clients in some way. Goal specification for social models of day care is often vaguely stated, and sometimes not stated at all. This may contribute to the fact that these programs often have difficulty getting adequately funded. In contrast, medical model day care programs are usually designed to provide services that qualify for third-party reimbursements for services to patients, and thus health-related goals are usually given priority. To the extent that these medical model programs provide the opportunity for caregiver respite, caregivers may be the targeted clients. But separate sources of funding must be found for any direct services for caregivers.

Sometimes the existing service system is targeted as being inadequate and for not providing needed services, and program goals are stated in terms of filling identified service gaps. This is frequently the case with funded demonstrations, such as the Medicare Alzheimer's Disease Demonstration, which supports the development of a variety of community-based services for persons with dementia and their caregivers. While it may be the intent of this program to eventually look for evidence that the program has impacted on the quality of life of elderly clients and their caregivers, implementation of this program and demonstration that it is meeting operational goals within the funding guidelines are still major considerations. Similarly, the Robert Wood Johnson Dementia Care and Respite Services Program is mainly asking their funded sites to demonstrate that they can provide and coordinate a variety of services in the community for persons with dementia and for their caregivers and charge reasonable fees that will eventually be sufficient to make the programs self-supporting.

Administrative and eligibility requirements may sometimes impose arbitrary program boundaries such that one program is considered respite and another is not, even though they are very similar in many respects. Interest group-based structures have provided models for the proliferation of specific disease-based programs, funding and eligibilities that are sometimes unnecessarily restricted. The types of relief and support provided to caregivers of terminal cancer patients by hospice programs are in many respects not unlike those provided by respite programs for Alzheimer's caregivers. It is often difficult to ascertain when the Alzheimers patients become "terminal," but their caregivers may be no less in need of more intense hospice-like support at this stage than are the caregivers of terminal cancer patients. Toseland and Rossiter (1989) found that the majority of support group intervention studies were for caregivers of Alzheimer's patients, but indicated they could find no evidence that the need for such interventions was any less for other caregivers. In fact, needs may be very similar for caregivers of persons with certain groups of diseases in which the risk of dementia is high, such as Parkinson's disease and stroke; but disease-based restrictions may fragment both services and recipients that might benefit from a broader base. Some have also argued that the biomedicalization of dementia has led us to emphasize the disease basis of behavior and to legitimize medical control over persons with dementing illnesses while neglecting social factors that may be just as important (Lyman 1989). From this perspective, respite programs might be seen as another aspect of "therapeutic nihilism" legitimated by the acceptance of progressive disease as the basis for behaviors that are stressful but unavoidable.

Respite program planners and administrators may have to designate clearly the number of hours provided and the frequency of care as well as the specific tasks to be performed in order to meet legal and reimbursement requirements. These requirements usually differentiate homemaker care from personal care, and the latter is often reimbursable when provided by a trained aide, ordered by a physician, and supervised by a nurse. However, the tasks required of the temporary substitute caregivers that respite care is providing may not fit neatly into the categories defined by these requirements. For example, the tasks required to care for someone with Alzheimer's disease usually vary with the stages or severity of dementia. Early on it may be sufficient to have someone who can come in and visit, look after, and help with meals and household routine. As the disease progresses and more personal care is needed, friends and volunteers may not be willing or able to provide the type of substitute care that is needed. If respite programs are meant to serve caregivers of persons at widely different stages of dementia, program goals and objectives may have to vary in accordance with these differences. Improving the quality of life of both caregivers and care-needing persons can be the overarching goal of these programs regardless of stage or severity of disease, but the problems that must be addressed and the specific outcomes that can be achieved may differ markedly. If the nature of the stress and burden associated with caring for persons with dementia in the community are pervasive, continuous and long-lasting, we should expect that temporary respite will, at best, provide temporary relief for caregivers. That is to say, caregivers may return to their caregiving after specific respite interventions more rested and with stress temporarily relieved, but the roles to which they return may continue to be stressful, upsetting and pervasive. It is not that caregivers, like conscientious workers, may take their stressful problems home with them at night. It is that they are at home with their stressful problems all day and all night. This suggests that the best time to collect evidence of the impact of respite is almost immediately after or even during each intervention rather than at the more remote times that characterize most studies.

In addition to the goals that are intentionally set, new and untested programs frequently have important unanticipated or unintended outcomes that are not recognized or are not adequately assessed. Sometimes these are desirable outcomes that could be incorporated as additional objectives or justifications for the programs. For example, it might turn out that persons who attend day care programs sleep better at night after a day full of activities and stimulation and that this provides their caregivers the opportunity for a full night of sleep. This may be as important to the quality of life of caregivers as the opportunity to get away from caregiving for a few hours during the day. However, there may be equally important outcomes that are undesirable. Patients might also return from day care agitated, restless and unable to sleep at night, and this could provide additional caregiving problems and stress. While respite programs are still in their early developmental periods, it is important that we are sensitive to the possibility that these programs may have important outcomes that are unanticipated and that we design our studies to take this possibility into consideration. Qualitative, descriptive and clinical evaluations of respite programs are especially able to identify outcomes such as these. More "scientific" quantitative and experimental evaluations are often constrained by the need to use more standardized and uniform measures of anticipated outcomes to test specific hypotheses, and they may miss entirely outcomes that are equally important. Both general types of research are needed in order to better understand the contributions that respite programs can realistically be expected to make.

Sometimes the outcomes of respite programs may serve to illustrate potentially conflicting goals. One of the unintended outcomes of respite care that has been noted is how it may smooth the transition from community caregiving to nursing home placement by legitimizing the need for institutional care and reducing the guilt of caregivers who have promised to keep their loved ones out of nursing homes. While this may result in improvement of the quality of life of primary caregivers, it may also result in shorter periods of community tenure (a possible reduction in the quality of life of the elderly person) and in higher costs associated with nursing home care. This illustrates how the goals of different parts of the system may be in potential conflict, and how the goals for different participants or even those of a single participant may conflict. The study conducted by the Office of Technology Assessment (OTA 1987) provides another illustration in reporting that while respite may postpone institutional placement, actual costs may be increased by the fact that persons whose admissions to institutions are delayed may need more expensive treatment services. Cost benefit analysis models have the potential for taking multiple outcomes such as these into consideration, but values and priorities need to be made explicit. There may be considerable disagreement over how to measure, value and prioritize quality-of-life related goals in such an analysis.

It follows from the above that evidence of goal attainment will differ considerably depending upon a wide variety of factors. At minimum these include (1) which goals are considered legitimate; (2) how restrictive or inclusive a definition of respite care is employed; (3) whether the patient, the caregiver or the long-term care system and other aspects of society are the intervention targets; (4) what aspects of the patient, the caregiver or the social system are addressed; (5) what special legal, administrative or reimbursement constraints, if any, apply; and (6) whether unanticipated or conflicting outcomes of intervention are also taken into consideration. Conspicuous among the important additional factors that are missing from this list are the technical and methodological issues that are regularly generated by research that attempts to ascertain whether programs have succeeded in achieving specific goals. The literature of evaluation research is replete with conflicting results and arguments over these issues, and research on whether the goals of respite programs have been attained is not immune from these problems. For example, Whitlatch, Zarat and von Eye (1991) have recently demonstrated that reanalysis of a study of the effects of intervention on caregivers of dementia patients yielded quite different results when different statistical techniques were employed.

If the goals of respite programs are social, they may range from simply filling what appear to be obvious gaps in the service provision system to reducing the use of nursing home beds. As far as gap-filling is concerned, the rapid increase in numbers of respite of programs, especially the state-supported ones, suggests that a serious and widespread effort is being made in this direction, but there is also considerable evidence that these services are still not widely available to many who express the need for them (George 1986; Fortinsky and Hathaway 1990). So far, we have not found any convincing evidence that there has been significant reduction in the use of nursing beds as a result of respite programs. However, as we have already indicated, if the usual, relatively restrictive definition of respite is used, reducing the use of nursing home beds does not appear to be an appropriate goal for such programs. Indeed, institutional-based short-stay respite programs might increase the use of nursing home beds intentionally in order to achieve quite different goals, and as noted earlier, community-based programs may result in earlier nursing home admissions for many persons.

It is worth pointing out that the goal of reducing the use of nursing home beds is similar in some respects to the goal of reducing the use of mental hospital beds that became popular about 25 years ago. Of course, many of the kinds of older persons who were once sent to mental hospitals now end up in nursing homes instead. In both situations many "reformers" have argued that the quality of life in the institutions was so poor that community-based alternatives had to be better. We now know that this is not true for many mental patients and for many older persons with dementia residing in the community. The economic motives behind the deinstitutionalization of mental patients were more subtly embedded in the early promises of psychotropic drugs than we now find among those arguing for less use of nursing home beds. However, psychotropic drugs have always been largely irrelevant as an argument for community care of the elderly, and a lack of serious efforts to provide better quality of life and better care in the community is shared by both these general attempts to reduce the use of institutions by the elderly. It is also worth noting that the kinds of community-based long-term care that could provide better quality of life for older persons with dementia, and possibly for their caregivers, are not respite programs, as we have defined them, nor are they necessarily less costly than nursing home care. For those who can afford to pay for it, home-based long-term care can often be found. In some communities, and especially in New York City during recent years, home-based long-term care is provided for many persons whose poverty is sufficient to qualify them for Medicaid. It is not clear whether these programs have reduced the use of nursing home beds, are less costly than nursing home beds, or provide a better quality of life than nursing homes.

Respite programs that target caregivers and those that target elderly dementia patients share many of the same problems. The goals they have set have often been unrealistic and inappropriate for the limited and short-term interventions that a relatively restrictive definition of respite would include. Hence studies that aim at determining whether depression or burden has been reduced among caregivers after a year or so of providing respite services will probably have disappointing results unless interventions not qualifying as respite under a relatively restricted definition are included. These too may have limited success, as intervention studies have shown (Toseland and Rossiter 1989; Montgomery and Bogata 1985; Lawton et al. 1989). These same studies tend to show that caregivers indicate they were very grateful for having received the services and that the quality of their lives was improved temporarily, but this may not provide sufficient basis for legislators to vote for public funding.

Hence economic considerations and structural factors will continue to push respite programs in the direction of services for cognitively impaired persons that are reimbursable and that can include respite to caregivers as an incidental indirect service. Where there is little or no public funding for programs that provide respite targeted for caregivers, existing programs will tend to depend more on volunteers or to charge substantial fees, and they will serve mostly white middle-class caregiving clients. Where there is substantial public funding for home care and related services available only under Medicaid, such programs will serve lower-income elderly persons who may have dementia but who are eligible to receive services for other reasons. These programs will tend to be found in more densely populated urban areas, and their clients will be disproportionately Black or Hispanic. Their caregivers may receive respite as a result of these services, but this may not even be a stated goal for the program. Hence there is no significant effort to gather evidence as to whether respite goals have been achieved for these groups. It is not an outcome that has been deemed important enough for data gathering. These types of definitional and boundary issues will continue to plague the gathering and interpreting of evidence about goal achievement of respite programs as long as the social context and structure of long-term care remain fragmented and irregular.

REFERENCES

Alzheimer's Disease and Related Disorders Association. *1990 Alzheimer's Association Directory of State Alzheimer's Programs and Legislation.* Chicago, ADRDA, 1990.

Fortinsky, R. and T.J. Hathaway. Information and service needs among active and former family caregivers of persons with Alzheimer's disease. *Gerontologist* 30:5, 1990.

George, L.K. Respite care: evaluating a strategy for easing caregiver burden. *Center Reports on Advances in Research* 10(2). Durham, NC: Center for the Study of Aging and Human Development, 1986.

Lawton, M.P., E.M. Brody and A.R. Saperstein. A controlled study of respite services for caregivers of Alzheimer's patients. *Gerontologist* 29(1):8-16, 1989.

Lyman, K.A. Bringing the social back in: a critique of the biomedicalization of dementia. *Gerontologist* 29(5):597-605, 1989.

Montgomery, R.J.V. and E.F. Bogata. *Family Support Project: Final Report to the Administration on Aging.* Seattle: University of Washington, 1989.

Montgomery, R.J.V. and E.F. Bogata. The effects of alternative support strategies on family caregiving. *Gerontologist* 29(4):457-464, 1989.

Office of Technology Assessment, U.S. Congress. *Losing a Million Minds: Confronting the Tragedy of Alzheimer's Disease and Other Dementias.* Washington, DC: U.S. Government Printing Office, 1989.

Reifler, B., H.R. Smyth and K. Sherrill. National dementia care and respite services program. *Generations,* Spring, 1990.

Seltzer, B., Y. Rheaume et al. The short-term effects of in-hospital respite on the patient with Alzheimer's disease. *Gerontologist* 28(1):121-124, 1988.

Toseland, R.W. and C.M. Rossiter. Group interventions to support family caregivers: a review and analysis. *Gerontologist* 29(4):438-448, 1989.

Vitaliano, P.P., H.M. Young and J. Russo. Burden: a review of measures used among caregivers of individuals with dementia. *Gerontologist* 31(1):67-75, 1991.

Weissert, W.G., J.M. Elston, E.J. Bolda et al. Models of adult day care: findings from a national survey. *Gerontologist* 29(5):640-649, 1989.

Whitlatch, C. J., S.H. Zarit and A. von Eye. Efficacy of interventions with caregivers: a reanalysis. *Gerontologist* 31(1):9-14, 1991.

Zarit, S.H. and R.W. Toseland. Current and future direction in family caregiving research. *Gerontologist* 29(4):481-483, 1989.